PERGAMON INTERNATIONAL LIBRARY
of Science, Technology, Engineering and Social Studies

*The 1000-volume original paperback library in aid of education,
industrial training and the enjoyment of leisure*

Publisher: Robert Maxwell, M.C.

LANGUAGE AND SPEECH DISORDERS IN CHILDREN

D0939477

THE PERGAMON TEXTBOOK
INSPECTION COPY SERVICE

An inspection copy of any book published in the Pergamon International Library
will gladly be sent to academic staff without obligation for their consideration for
course adoption or recommendation. Copies may be retained for a period of 60 days
from receipt and returned if not suitable. When a particular title is adopted or
recommended for adoption for class use and the recommendation results in a sale
of 12 or more copies the inspection copy may be retained with our compliments.
The Publishers will be pleased to receive suggestions for revised editions and new
titles to be published in this important international Library.

Pergamon Titles of Related Interest

Cartledge/Milburn TEACHING SOCIAL SKILLS TO CHILDREN: Innovative Approaches, Second Edition

Johnson/Rasbury/Siegel APPROACHES TO CHILD TREATMENT: Introduction to Theory, Research and Practice

Kirby/Grimley UNDERSTANDING AND TREATING ATTENTION DEFICIT DISORDER

Roberts PEDIATRIC PSYCHOLOGY: Psychological Interventions and Strategies for Pediatric Problems

Santostefano COGNITIVE CONTROL THERAPY WITH CHILDREN AND ADOLESCENTS

Related Journals
(Free sample copies available upon request)

CLINICAL PSYCHOLOGY REVIEW
JOURNAL OF CHILD PSYCHOLOGY AND PSYCHIATRY
JOURNAL OF SCHOOL PSYCHOLOGY

PSYCHOLOGY PRACTITIONER GUIDEBOOKS

EDITORS

Arnold P. Goldstein, Syracuse University
Leonard Krasner, SUNY at Stony Brook
Sol L. Garfield, Washington University

LANGUAGE AND SPEECH DISORDERS IN CHILDREN

JON EISENSON
Emeritus Professor, Hearing and Speech Science
Stanford University

PERGAMON PRESS
New York • Oxford • Beijing • Frankfurt
São Paulo • Sydney • Tokyo • Toronto

Pergamon Press Offices:

U.S.A.	Pergamon Press, Maxwell House, Fairview Park, Elmsford, New York 10523, U.S.A.
U.K.	Pergamon Press, Headington Hill Hall, Oxford OX3 0BW, England
PEOPLE'S REPUBLIC OF CHINA	Pergamon Press, Qianmen Hotel, Beijing, People's Republic of China
FEDERAL REPUBLIC OF GERMANY	Pergamon Press, Hammerweg 6, D-6242 Kronberg, Federal Republic of Germany
BRAZIL	Pergamon Editora, Rua Eça de Queiros, 346, CEP 04011, São Paulo, Brazil
AUSTRALIA	Pergamon Press (Aust.) Pty., P.O. Box 544, Potts Point, NSW 2011, Australia
JAPAN	Pergamon Press, 8th Floor, Matsuoka Central Building, 1-7-1 Nishishinjuku, Shinjuku-ku, Tokyo 160, Japan
CANADA	Pergamon Press Canada, Suite 104, 150 Consumers Road, Willowdale, Ontario M2J 1P9, Canada

---

First printing 1986

Library of Congress Cataloging in Publication Data

Eisenson, Jon, 1907-
    Language and speech disorders in children.

    (Psychology practitioner guidebooks)
    Bibliography: p.
    Includes index.
    1. Language disorders in children. 2. Speech
disorders in children. I. Title. II. Series.
[DNLM: 1. Language Disorders--in infancy & childhood.
2. Speech Disorders--in infancy & childhood.
WM 475 E36L]
RJ496.L35E37   1986   618.92′855   86-5070
ISBN 0-08-033182-3
ISBN 0-08-033181-5 (pbk.)

Printed in the United States of America

Contents

Preface

This guidebook on language and speech disorders in children is intended for professional practitioners—family physicians, pediatricians, nurse-practitioners, child psychologists, child psychiatrists, family counselors, and any other professional persons—who may be asked by a parent, "Is my child's speech normal?" To help answer this question, the practitioner will be provided with information about normal acquisition of speech and language (production and reception) by infants and young children, about indicators of slow and deviant development, and about significant abnormalities. The reader will also be provided information about when and to whom to make referrals for diagnosis and, if indicated, for treatment.*

The guidebook includes tables, charts, and checklists of motor and cognitive milestones that correlate with normal speech and language development from infancy through approximately 6 years of age. In addition, this guidebook covers the criteria for normalcy (from first cries to first sentences), articulation problems ("functional," neurological, and those associated with impaired hearing), hearing loss and its implications for language acquisition, brain damage and brain difference (frank cerebral palsy and "minimal brain dysfunction"), language delay, developmental aphasia, voice problems, stuttering, cluttering, and childhood autism.

---

*There is, of course, no reason to prevent parents from using this guidebook to answer their own questions about their children's speech.

Chapter 1
Is the Child's Speech Normal?

"Why isn't my child talking?" "Is there any reason why my child is so slow to talk?" "My boy is almost 2 years old; he speaks only two words we understand. Will he catch up and have normal speech? He seems to understand what we say, but can't make himself understood except when he points. Then we guess."

As a psychologist specializing in language problems, these are questions I am asked almost every working day. The questions are almost always from anxious and concerned parents, and more often about boys than girls. Usually, the parents had been told by someone they respected—their pediatrician or family doctor—that their youngster's speech was abnormally delayed or that the child was "not talking right"; sometimes, the impetus came from a relative who could not be ignored. The observation that something about the child's speech was not right often confirmed the parent's own concerned impression. On occasion, parents would consult me months after they had seen a pediatrician and had been assured that there was no cause to worry. "Be patient; many children do not talk until almost 3 years of age." But their child was now uncomfortably close to that age, and they saw no progress in intelligible speech. However, these particular parents knew that the child understood them, unless they spoke too fast or tried to say too much at one time.

In my interviews with parents I usually open with, "Tell me, what is there about your child's speech that brings us together in my office?"

The most frequent reply is, "Johnny (or Joannie) isn't talking right."

"Try to be specific," I usually say. "Give me some examples of what Johnny says, or fails to say, or what you expect him to say. If you can, say it just the way he does."

I may then get a description of "baby talk" or of hesitant, repetitive speech that parents are likely to call stuttering or stammering. Occasional-

1

ly, parents explain, "Bobby seems to talk a blue streak, but we can't make head or tail of what he is trying to say. It's a lot of jargon. When we don't understand, he throws a temper tantrum or just gives up trying. Sometimes he cries in frustration. Sometimes we cry along with him."

Sometimes, but much less frequently, parents tell me, "Mary was born brain damaged. She's 4 years old but doesn't talk. Often, she doesn't understand what we say. Will Mary ever talk? What can we do for her?"

Sometimes I am informed, "Karen has a cleft palate. She talks, but we often have difficulty in understanding her. When she has a cold, she has difficulty in understanding us. Can she be helped?"

Perhaps the most frequent complaint of parents is, "Billy is late in talking. He is 2 years old and only says about five or six words that we understand. His sister was talking almost like a grown-up when she was Billy's age."

All the questions raised by the parents, and their answers to my questions, show proper and usually justified concern. In essence, they are asking, "Is my child's speech normal?" or "Why isn't our child talking?" or "Is there any reason to believe that our child will not be talking right?" or "What can we do to help our child talk right?" When such questions are addressed to a pediatrician, a family doctor, a child psychologist, a child psychiatrist, or a specialist in speech and language, the parents have a right to replies that are neither put-offs nor put-downs. All too often they hear, "Don't worry, your child will outgrow it." This is the wrong answer.

In a majority of cases, in my interviews and follow-up sessions, I have been able to reassure parents that nothing was significantly wrong with their child's speech that time and growing a little bit older would not cure. In some instances, I recommend assistance from a speech therapist or a language clinician. Occasionally, I feel the need to recommend help from a child psychiatrist or child psychologist to get at the problem behind the immediate problem: the complaint about the child's speech. On occasion, I recommend counseling for the parents (note the plural). Every so often I suggest speech or voice therapy for one or both of the parents as well as for the child.

In my sessions with parents, I ask many questions about the child's early health history, the child's early crying and play sounds, the child's responses to sounds: human, animal, and mechanical. I ask about age of walking, left-, right-, or neither-handedness, how the child keeps himself or herself occupied when awake, who talks to the child, and what happens when the child tries to talk. But the most frequent questions I ask are "Does the child pay attention to you when you talk directly to him (or her)?" "Does the child understand you?" "How do you know?"

These are significant questions that will be explained and answered in detail in later chapters of this book. But an early explanation is in order.

WHAT IS NORMAL?

In a strict sense, the first question, "Is my child's speech normal?" should refer only to a youngster who is already talking. But children tell us a great deal about their potential as speakers before they say their first recognizable words. They tell us about themselves in their early crying, and in their cooing, gurgling, and babbling. The sounds they make before they talk are their own prologue to their future talking.

We can begin to appreciate how much children understand of what we say to them by their actions 3–6 months before they say their first words. Note that we are using a range of time. "Normal" is not a point but a period or range. *"Within certain limits" is normal.* Just beyond these limits is near normal. Normal is about right—it is rarely exactly right.

We need to keep in mind that no human being of any age is always the same degree of normal. Even within a range, the term "normal" only tells us about the child's behavior at the time we make our judgment. Some children start late and catch up. These by far outnumber the few children who start early and fall behind. (These few probably had something happen to them—illness, accident, or adjustment problems—that spoiled the promise of an early start.)

With the basic understanding that "normal" is a range, not a certain age or time or a specific accomplishment, we can provide at least tentative answers to parents' questions. Most of these questions center around three main points: *Articulation*—How well has my child mastered the sounds of the language system? *Vocabulary*—Is his or her vocabulary large enough to indicate needs, feelings, and thoughts? *Syntax*—Is my child proficient in putting words together according to the rules (grammar) of the language?*

In recent years, authorities in speech and language development have made several observations regarding these questions. These findings have important and broad implications. Here are a few of them:

A child should begin to understand some of the things said to him or her on repeated occasions between the ages of 6 and 9 months, unless deaf, severely hard of hearing, or mentally retarded. The child may show understand-

---

*The term *speech*, for the present, will be confined to the production of the sounds of a language system and accompanying vocalization or phonation. *Language* refers to the content (the vocabulary and syntax or grammar) that carries the meanings (semantics) of a symbol-language system. The two systems, speech and language, are obviously intimately related.

ing by behavior as simple as a change in position, such as getting ready to be picked up when mother says, "Up baby," or "Come baby, up," or "Up we go," and the like. This child should change position when the words alone are spoken, even before or without the picking-up gestures of the mother. Similarly, the child may offer a hand on the request, "Give me your hand, darling," or look expectantly for father if mother says, "Here comes daddy."

Most children who are going to talk, perhaps up to 90% of them, say their first words by 15 months. Some say their first words as early as 9 months, and a few precocious ones (who are more likely to be girls than boys) as early as 8 months.

The first words need not be of adult form. Any sound combination produced fairly regularly to identify (or label) a person, thing, or event is acceptable as a first word. So *wawa* will do for water, and *doddy* or *goggi* for doggy, or *buh-buh* for daddy. Mothers, happily, are more likely to be called *mama*, or something very close to it, than fathers are to be called *dada*. When a child is beginning to talk, it is he or she who determines the form of the word, not the adult.

Within a month or two after a child has begun to build up a naming or labeling vocabulary, he or she is likely to begin using some of these words to make things happen. The child uses words as tools to bring things about, in addition to using them as labels for what is present or happening. Words now are the forerunners of events, as well as the names of objects or persons the child wants. So the child will call "mommy" when mother is wanted, or announce "wawa" to get a drink, or demand "doddy" to get the doll or the stuffed animal, or even shout "up" to be picked up.

By the time a child has a vocabulary of about 50-60 words as labels or as demands, he or she usually begins to combine them into two-word "statements." For most children, this occurs by 18 months. These "statements" or infant sentences are likely to take the form of *baby up* or *baby wawa* or *baby mama*. Each statement indicates what the child wants and expects to happen as a result of his or her announcement.

The child's comprehension of language exceeds the child's ability to speak. This is so, of course, for the rest of any individual's life. We all understand more words than we use.

These five guideposts should help relieve parental anxiety and offer basic answers to the question, "Is my child's speech normal?" Later I will provide other answers, in greater detail, about degrees of normality, about apparently different children who should still be no cause for concern, and about other children for whom there should be not only concern but also action to reduce what might otherwise become a serious delay in talking, thinking, and learning.

EACH CHILD IS AN INDIVIDUAL

Everyone has an individual way of speaking—including young children. By the time a child is 4 years old, he or she speaks with the language of the surrounding grown-ups, using the words and grammar of the grown-ups, but still manages to speak in a distinctive way. Each child learns words, the words of older speakers with whom he or she has contact, yet also has favorite words and favorite ways of turning a phrase, of making statements and asking questions. Although a normal human being shows the influence of others, no individual is a replica of any other human being. In regard to language, every normal child somehow figures out sounds and words, and the rules that govern sounds and words, and becomes a speaker of his or her own native language. Yet the child also speaks the language in an individual manner that is adapted to the occasion.

Human beings are supposed to talk. Psychologists, anthropologists, and others who qualify as authorities on the matter of talking sum up their observations on the subject in a variety of technical terms. But, in simplest form, their findings come down to "Human beings talk." That, as a minimum, is what it means to be human. Of course, we know that *some* human beings *do not* talk. We also know that those who do talk vary considerably in this distinctive achievement.

Why some children do not talk, and why some who do talk begin so late in their young lives as to cause anxiety in parents (and grandparents), we will consider in some detail in later chapters of this book. There are reasons for late onset of talking, for slowness in understanding speech, for defective speech, and for absence of speech.

Beginning with the birth cry, numerous signs reveal whether or when a child will begin to talk—and, to an important degree, how capable or at least how close to normal he or she will be in early talking. This is not to say that we can make predictions with absolute certainty; we need to leave a margin for error in our estimates. But the margin is not great. We now know considerably more about how children acquire their language than we did in the 1950s and 1960s. A professional person responsible for providing guidance to parents about their children should know whereof he or she speaks when telling parents, for example, "Don't worry, everything will be all right. I have known children who didn't begin to talk until they were 3 years old.

To be sure, there are early talkers and late talkers; but mere chance is not the determining factor. Age 3 is late to begin talking. It *is* exceptional for a child to be a late talker in a family of early talkers, or to be an early talker in a family that includes late talkers on both the mother's and father's side. Of course, the early talker is not likely to cause concern to parents. But the exceptionally late talker may, quite legitimately, be a cause for concern—not only to his parents but also to the professional advisor.

HELP FOR CHILDREN
WITH PROBLEMS

In later chapters, I shall consider the normal development of speech in great detail. I shall offer advice about what parents can do to enhance their children's acquisition of speech, and what they should avoid doing—when "lay off" is the best policy but also when "it's time to get going." I shall also describe children who are conspicuously late in talking and some who may never achieve more than a modicum of speech. We shall consider problems such as cluttering and stuttering, deviant articulation, defective voice production, and the special problems of children with severe hearing loss and those with impaired physical apparatus for speaking. We shall consider the child, and the parents of the child, who has difficulty relating to other human beings and does not talk, or who responds with considerable delay to a speaker, with a delayed echo, or who uses stereotyped words or phrases that seem to be unrelated to the occasion.

The Professional Speech-Language
Pathologists and Audiologists

Speech pathologists (I prefer to identify them as speech and language clinicians) are specialists who usually hold a degree at the master's or doctoral level. Their areas of expertise are in the diagnosis and treatment of speech and language problems that may be congenital (developmental) or acquired as a result of illness or injury. In some areas of the United States, and often in schools, the term *speech correctionist* is used synonymously with speech pathologist or speech clinician.

Audiologists are specialists in hearing, both normal and defective. They are concerned with the measurement of hearing, the identification of hearing loss, and the treatment to improve effectiveness of hearing in persons with hearing loss.

Teachers of the deaf are educational specialists who work with deaf children, usually in schools.

These professionals function in a variety of settings. Most of these professionals are employed in public elementary and secondary schools. They may be self-employed or may work in medical settings or in college and university clinics that have academic training programs. Many are employed in agencies operated by the Easter Seal Society or by the United

Cerebral Palsy Association. In Canada, the Elks Purple Cross Fund supports training programs and treatment clinics.

In the United States, their professional organization is the American Speech-Language-Hearing Association (ASHA). This association publishes several journals, maintains standards, and evaluates and certifies candidates for their professional competence in speech pathology and audiology. Many states have organizations that follow ASHA guidelines for certification. Canada and England have comparable national and regional organizations.

Chapter 2
First Cries to First Words

The sounds made by infants, from birth cries to vocal play, are precursors and often prognosticators of their first stages of speech production. Comparably, an infant's responses to sounds, both human and nonhuman (environmental), are indicators of the child's ability to comprehend spoken language. In a broad sense, both aspects, responses and early production of sounds, are components of the processes that culminate in the comprehension and production of spoken language.

There is an increasing recent awareness of a likely continuity between early sound making and listening (responding to sounds); that infants progress from reflexive sound making to intentional sound making, first in their crying and later in their speaking. What infants do, how they respond, is an important prognosticator of later speech and language development, and they are actively involved in using sounds to communicate with their caretakers. They initiate cooing and babbling not just for play but to obtain and maintain attention and interest from older persons. In brief, normal infants are involved and determined sound makers almost from the beginning of their lives.

INFANT CRYING

When in pain or discomfort, all of God's creatures who are capable of making noise do so. Children are no exception. The way children cry tells us how they are: whether all is going well or whether conditions need correcting. One condition for the infant in the first month of life may be that the infant is not breathing properly or needs some help to get going. Or the baby may simply need something to fill his or her tummy, or burping, or a change of linen, or merely a change of position in the crib. Rarely does a baby cry without reason.

We affirm this despite what parents, grandparents, and especially neighbors may say to the contrary. Unfortunately, a baby cannot explain the crying. A child who is old enough to provide reasons usually doesn't need to resort to crying. If crying persists, it shows that the child has somehow learned that crying is more effective than talking in getting one's way, or in getting rid of what is not wanted.

How should babies cry? Lustily and loudly, and long enough to show they mean it. That kind of crying indicates that physiologically, at least, all is well. The doctor who delivers the baby may have to give a sharp whack on the backside to get the infant breathing—and so the child begins to cry. The newborn infant, no matter what cynical philosophers may say, does not intend to cry. Babies cry because they cannot help themselves. For the moment, it hurts to have to breathe on one's own. It hurts because mother-warmed vocal cords have become a bit chilled now that the baby has left the protection of the mother's body. The infant cries because the change in climate, in his or her new environment, suddenly causes the vocal cords to contract. As the newborn gasps for air, the vocal cords are set in motion. This, too, hurts a bit, so the infant cries. The baby is responding purely reflexively to all the sudden changes in his or her life.

Normal babies cry much alike. A characteristic cry—a good cry—usually has three identifiable phases. In phase one, the baby seems to be tentative about vocalization. He or she appears to be trying out the mechanism and his or her intention by a whimper or two. The infant is tuning up, preparing for the next phase.

In the second phase, the baby goes all out, perhaps because the baby has been frightened with the intensity of his or her behavior. A just audible *wa-wa* or *naa-naa* or *ai-ai*, or a variety of such sounds, increases to a loud crescendo that may change from a low pitch to a high one. After this, the infant may pause for just a moment and then start over again. And again. And yet again.

In the third phase, the baby sounds as though he or she is petering out, at least for the time being. And the baby may well be finished, if the parent or other caretaker changes whatever caused the crying in the first place. If the discomfort has not been eased, perhaps because the caretaker didn't guess correctly what was needed, the crying will be resumed. The third phase may well be a warning that means, "I'm putting you on alert. Do what is necessary to make me comfortable. If you don't, there's more where that came from."

If the baby cries in these three stages and gives you the message, "I'm about to cry, I'm crying, I'm about to stop but I can go at it again," the caretaker has reason to be grateful. The baby is making a good start toward becoming a normal talker. The baby's first crying sounds, like most first activities, are spasmodic and not under control. They are reflexive and, in a very real sense, they control the child. If you observe what is taking place when a baby cries, you will probably note that the baby's crying beyond phase one is a total body affair. The entire body is at work, legs and arms in motion, facial muscles contracted. Literally, the infant is crying all over.

What of the baby who cries with a mere whimper and then stops? What of the "good baby" who rarely ever cries and seems content to be alone, even when awake? These babies will be considered later. At the present time, I will only suggest that babies *should* cry, that normal babies *do* cry, and that almost all of them do so in the manner described. If the baby cries too little, or too much, or merely whimpers in a token manner, consult the pediatrician or family physician. Parents have a right to be assured that all is well, or to be informed of what they should do if all is not well.

Assuming that the baby is born full term and that everything goes smoothly, we can anticipate changes in crying after the first 3 or 4 weeks. During the first few weeks, the baby cries with a limited repertoire of sounds. He or she is usually a virtuoso only in regard to loudness. When hungry, the infant may combine loud volume and pitch in a rhythmic production that accompanies the contractions and relaxations of an empty tummy. All we can guess from the baby's vocal performance other than the hunger cry is that he or she is uncomfortable or in actual pain. But, otherwise, the crying is uninformative and not even a loving mother or a doting grandmother can do anything but guess at the cause of the discomfort. A need for a change of linen is a likely exception, because it may stimulate senses other than hearing in the observer.

Compared to normal children born full term, brain-damaged infants may cry excessively and cannot be comforted as readily once their crying is under way. Bosma (1975) notes:

> The cry of an infant at term is composed of stably balanced elements that are characteristic of the individual infant. Appropriate to this interindividual heterogeneity, the range of normal variation is great. (pp. 471–472)

He also observes:

> Crying differs from developing speech in its occasion of stress and arousal, in the associated exclusion responses to incidental stimuli, and in its stability of performance pattern. In the young infant, crying may be reciprocal to the prologues of early speech. (p. 475)

Despite individual variations in their patterns of crying, most normal infants cry with identifiable patterns that serve to distinguish them from those who are brain damaged or are at high risk for abnormalities associated with prematurity, from children who have Down's syndrome, or from those who may later be identified as having primary autism. Some of these cry-pattern differences are described by Karelitz and Fischelli (1962), Truby, Bosma, and Lind (1966), and Wasz-Hockert, Lind, Vourenkoski, Partanen, and Valanne (1968).

Discomfort and Comfort Sounds:
Crying and Cooing

Beginning with the second month, the baby can express considerably more by crying than he or she did as a newborn. Part of the baby's waking time is spent in making sounds that fond parents refer to as *cooing*. Though some of the sounds do resemble the cooing of the dove, most are more varied and more interesting. In an important way, the sounds of the cooing stage seem to be under the baby's control. In the first 4 weeks, the occasional grunting and gurgling noises sound like by-products of digestive activity. (Perhaps that is why Shakespeare referred to the infants as "mewling and puking in the nurse's arms.") But beginning in the second month the baby who had the benefit of a full-term pregnancy and a normal delivery makes sounds to signal that all is well in the world. The infant also makes considerably more vehement and strident sounds to signal that all is *not* well. Some of these discomfort sounds are now sufficiently different from one another to convey what is wrong. Now, the hunger cry is different from the gas-in-the-tummy cry and from the cry that ceases when the baby is turned over, or has his or her linen changed, or has the bed coverings rearranged to give room for arms and legs to move.

In a very important way, both the crying and the cooing tell parents something about their baby's state of being. Though the baby's sound making is still reflexive, without conscious intent, the child is nevertheless sending informative signals. These signals, because they are different from each other, reduce the amount of guessing that the baby's parents need to do. The baby now has the important beginnings of communication.

One of the things the baby's crying and cooing tell us is how the baby is feeling about himself or herself while vocalizing. This component of the message will continue throughout life. By our tone of voice, by the way we sound, we reveal how we truly feel about what we say. Just as our words tell what we are thinking, our voice tells how we feel about the thoughts we are sharing. It takes the skill of an accomplished actor or a thoroughly practiced liar to make the voice conceal rather than reveal our feelings. The infant's vocalizations are sincere: his or her voice reflects and reveals current feelings to the sympathetic listener.

Cooing: The Comfort Sounds

What do the comfort sounds, the so-called *cooings*, tell us? Can we really describe these sounds? It is easier to answer the first question than the second. For one thing, comfort sounds tell us that the infant is a sound maker capable of revealing that "I'm O.K." as well as "I need help to become O.K." The comfort sounds also tell us that the child is maturing, that the child has the neurological and physical equipment to reveal his or her general state of being. The baby is capable, even though not yet aware of it, of communicating broad-based messages to those who will listen. And, if those who listen respond, the capability will be encouraged and nurtured, and the child will mature.

The specific names we give to the sounds of cooing (the non-crying sounds produced while content) depend as much on our subjective attitude as on the actual sounds the infant makes. According to who is listening and doing the naming, the baby may be said to grunt or gurgle, to hiccough or cluck, to babble or bubble, to coo, snort, squeal, and/or to breathe heavily with accompanying vocal noise.

What the infant produces is a result of how she or he feels, a reflexive by-product of the physiological state. However, *how much* and for how long the infant vocalizes is likely to be positively related to the amount of attention and response the infant receives when making sounds. A "nonverbal dialogue," or even a verbal one if the caretaker responds in words, has a positive influence on the child's sound making. Conversely, the ignored child may cease cooing and give way to crying to establish a "dialogue" and then resume nonverbal production. In effect, unless the child is colicky,* the parent or other caretaker has considerable influence over the infant's early, as well as later, sound making.

Those of us who speak English or American English are likely to identify several English vowels and a few English consonants in a baby's crying or cooing vocabulary. The vowels most frequently identified (many others are heard but not identified or remembered) include the long *e* as in *knee*, *i* as in *it*, *e* as in *wet*, and the *a* of *hat*. All these sounds are produced with the front of the tongue, arched and active. Phoneticians (experts in the sound patterns of a language) call them *front vowels*. Interestingly, the baby is not likely to produce the long *oo* as in *coo* until he or she is 3 or 4 months of age.

Another note of interest is that vowel sounds produced in a state of comfort have little or no nasal quality. This is likely to be so even for French-speaking children of French-speaking parents who use nasal reinforcement (speak "through the nose") much more than most speakers of English. English-speaking cultures associate "talking through the nose" with whining and unpleasant states. We may observe that in our culture, children express pleasantness with oral reinforcement while discontent-

---

*In his book, *Crybabies*, Weissbluth (1984, p. 13) defines colic as "inconsolable crying for which no physical cause can be found, which lasts more than 3 hours a day, occurs at least 3 days a week and continues for at least 3 weeks."

ment is reinforced "by the trombone of the nose." Playing these different tones and varied tunes on a conscious and controlled level is something that the child must learn to do. But from 1 month of age to 3 or 4 months, the tunes come naturally, spontaneously, and sincerely.

Normal and Abnormal Early Infant Sounds

The following summary statements of infant cries may help differentiate the sounds made by normal children from those of potentially abnormal children and serve as guides for future speech development.*

A typical *birth cry* is 1 second long and is usually produced on a rising-falling pattern. In a normal sequence, the baby takes one or two gasping inspirations and then produces the cry. The pattern is repeated.

A *hunger cry* typically has its own sequence: a cry, a brief silence (rest), followed by a quick inspiration "whistle," and another rest, then repetition of the sequence.

A *pain cry* is, in general, similar to the hunger crying sequence. Turbulence results from the forcing of excess breath through the vocal bands. The cry is then likely to be louder, noisier, and has more interruptions and gagging than the response to hunger (see Figure 2.1).

Pleasure "cries" (cooing) do not usually resemble the sound making of doves. When the infant is content, vocal productions may show rises and falls in pitch and include grunts, gurgles, hiccoughs, clucks, babble, snorts, squeals, heavy breathing and, occasionally, sounds that suggest cooing.

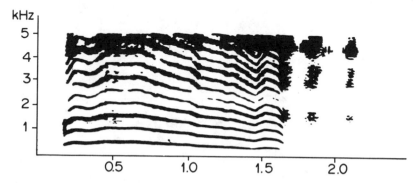

FIGURE 2.1. Pain cry of a healthy newborn baby. *Note.* From *Infant Communication* (2nd ed.), (p. 138) by T. Murry and J. Murry, 1980, San Diego: College Hill Press. Copyright 1980 by College Hill Press. Used with permission.

---

*The basic source for most of these statements is Wasz-Hockert et al., 1968.

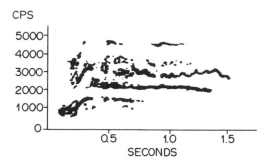

FIGURE 2.2. Pain cry from a baby (2 days old) with clinical diagnosis of asphyxia neonatorum and brain damage. Note the double phonation at 0.7 and 1.4 seconds. *Note.* Figures 2.2, 2.3 and 2.4 are from *The Infant Cry* by O. Wasz-Hockert et al., 1968, London: Spastics International Medical Publications. Copyright 1968 by Mac Keith Press. Used with permission.

Abnormal cries vary considerably from the patterns described above. Some deviant patterns follow:

Abnormal pain cries are not well sustained and are often produced with double phonation (see the spectograms in Figures 2.2 and 2.3).

A *Down's syndrome* child's cry is usually weaker than a normal cry and is likely to be breathy and double-toned (see Figure 2.4).

An *autistic child's cry* is likely to be weak and poorly sustained. Many autistic children are silent, some almost to the point of mutism. The absence of crying explains the parents' identification of autistic children as ''good babies.''

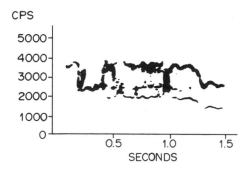

FIGURE 2.3. The same baby pictured in Figure 2.2 at 3 days old. The cry has different features, but the double phonation is still present.

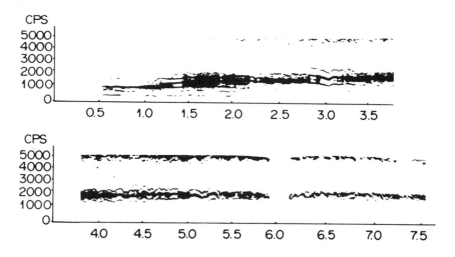

FIGURE 2.4. Pain cry of a baby with Down's syndrome.

The *cri du chat* (cry of a cat) is an unusual cry of an unusual child. Presumably, because the infant is born with a small and weak larynx, the cry is high pitched and mewling. Subjectively, it is a painful cry for the listener as well as the infant. Cri du chat children lack chromosome 5 (see Figure 2.5).

Table 2.1 summarizes the prelanguage vocal responses of normal infants. Details of the developmental sequence follow.

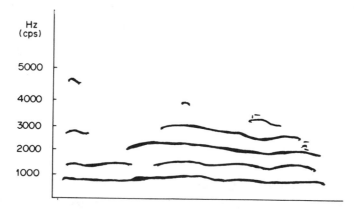

FIGURE 2.5. Characteristic features of the cry of "cri du chat" syndrome. *Note.* Adapted from Wasz-Hockert et al. (1968), Ostwald and Peltzman (1974), and Murry and Murry (1980).

Table 2.1. Early Vocal Responses and Producations Before First Words

Approximate Age	Baby Hears or Sees	Baby Responds
Birth–2 Months	Loud noise	Cries
	Baby cries	Cries
	Eye contact with adult	Coos
	Self-initiated (reflexive) sounds	Reflexively yawns, gurgles, coughs, sneezes, coos when content; may produce sounds such as *ayruh* when distressed.
2 Months	Angry voice	Baby cries and may turn away from voice (vocalizer).
	Nonangry voice	If crying, may stop. May coo in response.
2–3 Months	Sees face or hears familiar voice	Chuckling noise; laughter
	Unpleasant voice	Cries
4–5 Months	Social play with adult; tickling	Laughter, as for an older child, "singing" (cooing) when child is alone and content.
6 Months	Speaking person	Variety of vocal responses to indicate feelings; may "exclaim" to show delight; child responds to differences in vocal melody (intonation) patterns. Babbles.
7–9 Months	Speaking person	Child's vocal contours (melody-intonation) suggest requests, demands; sophisticated cooing expresses calmness and contentment. May say first words.
10 Months	Adult voice (speaking person)	Child responds by adjusting own pitch level in direction of the voice pitch of the adult; higher when responding to woman than to man. First words to identify (label) events.

Data adapted from Lieberman (1966); Lewis (1951); Renfrew and Murphy (1964); and P. H. Wolff in Foss (1966).

Babbling

Two or three months after becoming a part-time-awake-but-non-crying sound maker, the child is likely to begin true *babbling*. Now the child, usually by 16 to 20 weeks of age, seems to be listening to the sounds produced and may repeat a few of them. If we view this behavior generously, we may note that the child occasionally smiles or makes an approving gurgling noise after one of these renditions. Sometimes, such divinely inspired oral renditions take place just before the baby falls asleep, and so the parents are likely to miss them.

Babbling in the early stages is very much a private affair. Babbling, or any other form of sound making for that matter, is likely to be interrupted by the intrusion of another sound maker. Unfortunately, babbling is likely to stop altogether if interrupted, while crying is only momentarily impeded.

But after the child has practiced babbling for a month or two, the presence of another babbler may result in a social dialogue rather than silence or crying. The second participant, however, must be careful not to overwhelm the baby with a flood of oral noises. Gently and easily is the way if babbling is to be encouraged. Incidentally, each babbler says his or her own thing. Each encourages the other, but the sounds and the "music" are unrelated.

After beginning to babble (producing repetitive or near-repetitive sounds and syllables) the child may still resort to cooing. Babies do not entirely give up the behavior of an early stage when they advance to a new one. They can always "regress" to an earlier stage, according to their needs. Normally, babbling, as a new and identifiable stage, and later self-repetitive imitation (lalling) lasts until 6 to 8 months of age.

Lalling is speech sound repetition. Babbling tells us that the child has the necessary equipment to make speech sounds and that making a variety of sounds is fun. Lalling—the repetition of sounds that initiate with the child, such as *la-la-la, da-da-da,* or *na-na-na,* tells us that the child not only enjoys sound making but that he or she can hear the sounds made and can control (repeat) them. The child is in control of his or her productions and finds this achievement good.

Many parents wonder, however, whether their baby really is hearing voices and other noises in a normal way. Perhaps their baby is unusually quiet or unresponsive when spoken to. How can concerned parents tell whether there is a real hearing problem? And if there seems to be one, what can they do about it?

Deaf or hearing-impaired children (for no child is completely without hearing) begin to babble at about the same age and under the same conditions as children who hear normally. Moreover, they sound much the same as normal babies. By the end of the fifth or sixth month, however, the deaf baby makes fewer sounds than the hearing child. Both the quantity and the variety of babbling are considerably less in deaf babies than in normal ones. Moreover, the deaf child's babblings are self-started. He or she does not engage in dialogues, nor does the deaf infant respond to another babbler.

Presumably, deaf children are quieter because they lack the normal and adequate feedback that comes from hearing their own speech and that of others. The feedback obtained by feeling the movements of the tongue and lips is ordinarily not enough to maintain babbling or start lalling. In the absence of the ability to hear as well as feel the sounds they produce, they tend to become silent children, unless they are made to feel uncomfortable. Even then, the sounds they produce are likely to be those made in the early babbling period, with a flat and nasal quality.

But babbling is very important, even for the hard-of-hearing (those with moderately impaired hearing). Eventually the child will learn to speak, and his or her speaking apparatus needs to be kept in "good running order." Babbling needs to be encouraged. This is a special problem with the child suspected of having a severe hearing loss. It should be referred to a clinician who has the authority born of knowledge and experience with young children.

In addition, parents can encourage their baby's babbling by arranging a mirror or mirrors above the crib. Then the baby can not only feel but also see himself or herself talking, and the babbling is not only encouraged but also sustained and possibly prolonged. The infant keeps the apparatus for sound making in good shape. To the limits of his or her hearing, the baby is also *practicing listening*.

The babbling–lalling stage is extremely important to all speech development, from its beginning as a self-initiated "private affair" on through subsequent stages into social dialogue. Parents and other caretakers can encourage this normal sequence by controlled participation. They should not overwhelm the baby by a torrential flow of vocalization. They, and the baby, should wait and take turns so that the monologues may become dialogues. Babbling and, later, lalling indicate that the infant has a working feedback system and that all is probably going well with speech development, with listening as well as producing sounds that will soon become incorporated or shaped into spoken language.

Differences in Vocalization Between Normal Infants and Those Likely to be Delayed in Speech

Evidence that the child is "tuning in" to his or her caretakers, the influential sound makers, is revealed in vocalizations produced as early as 6 weeks of age. Discerning adults may note that normal infants begin to produce speechlike sounds in their babbling and increase such sound making as they grow older. Normal hearing infants also begin to imitate the intonation patterns of adult speech as early as 6 months. In contrast, deaf infants usually continue in their babbling (self-initiated, reflexive) without speechlike sounds (Maskarinec, Cairns, Butterfield, & Weamer, 1981).

Differences are also found in the amount of time devoted to sound play. Normal infants increase sound play; the deaf do not. Retarded children, on the whole, start sound play at a later age than normal infants and continue in the early babbling stage for a longer time without evidence of self-imitation (lalling). Autistic infants rarely engage in sound play and almost never in socialized vocalization.

Sound Imitation: The Echoic Stage

Beginning at about 8 months—the range may be from 7 to 9 or even 10 months—most children begin to imitate some of the sounds and even short words they hear other people making. Lalling and even babbling, both self-initiated, are of course likely to continue. In the echoic stage the child *sounds as if he or she is talking.* If mother says "mama" or "baby," the child responds with either a remarkable imitation or one very close to the target. At this stage, the baby has a real capacity for echoing what he or she hears, or at least part of it. However, though the child may utter "ma-ma" or "da-da" or even "bye-bye," the child probably doesn't mean what he or she seems to be saying. The child does not indicate *mama* is meant by looking at her, nor does the child look in the direction through which mama is likely to enter the room. If the baby's actions were appropriate for the echoic words, the child would then be speaking. He or she would be using verbal labels for one or two somebodies, or one or two things. But that is the next stage of speech development.

Although the child is not yet speaking—truly speaking—he or she is learning to listen to and understand the language spoken in his or her immediate environment. He or she does respond to some names and even to some directions when others speak, and will turn to mother, to daddy, to a doll, or to a teddy bear on hearing the appropriate name. The child will get ready to be picked up, provided of course that he or she is in the mood for this activity, when mother or daddy or another trusted adult says "up" or "up baby." The child may hug a favorite doll when that is suggested, or may reach out when asked, "Do you want your doll?" Probably the child is responding to a key word of the statement or question, but at the same time is responding and building up his or her comprehension vocabulary. The child is involved in the game of language!

FIRST WORDS

"Hi" or "bye-bye," accompanied by appropriate gestures, are likely to be the first "words" of most normal, socialized children. These social gesture "words" are, in fact, part of the process and proof of the infant's socialization. *Mama* and *dada, more,* and *up* are other early words that may be used for social interaction before they may begin to be used as references (naming or labeling).

By the end of the first year, some children, more often girls than boys, evoke their first naming-labeling words. Most of these are likely to be references to person, animals, or objects; some, such as *up* and *more* may be used to identify or even to initiate an activity or to keep a pleasant one going.

Most children, and especially most boys, arrive at the identification or labeling stage by 15 months of age. Some do not get there until 18 to 20 months. A few may torment their parents and grandparents by holding back until they are age 2 or even 2½ years old. I know a boy whose parents are both professionals, and who did not begin to talk until he was almost 3½ years of age. However, there was no reason to doubt his ability to hear and understand what was said to him, and a good deal of what was said about him. This is exceptional. Equally exceptional was that at age 14 he was admitted to college, graduated at age 17, and at age 21, had a medical degree. At age 25 he completed his medical residence in psychiatry. So, one can never be sure how a late talker is going to turn out.

Children who speak normally usually begin to show that they understand spoken language addressed directly to them by 9 months of age, a few as early as 6 or 7 months. This language is usually a polite "command" or direction such as "open your mouth" or "give me your hand." By 2 years of age the great majority of children who will be normal speakers have begun speaking. Some begin about 9 months; most begin by 15 months. Notice—and this is a very important point—that there are two parts to the language game, *understanding* and *speaking*. The child who says only a few words but understands many words should be no cause for concern, even at 2½ years of age.

Late Speakers

If the child understands what is said there is less cause for concern than if the child neither understands nor talks. But even if the child understands speech, there is reason for *concern* and *action* if the child is not talking by 3 years of age.

Why some children start early and others start late is not yet clear. There is a tendency for the age of onset of talking to run in families. When the tendencies run the same on both sides of the family, we are likely to have less anxiety than when mother's side has early talkers and daddy's side is somewhat slower. Later, especially in Chapter 8, I shall go into factors that are related to the onset of talking.

The late-speaking child who is from a family of early speakers (especially if late to understand speech) needs to be considered differently from the late-speaking or even nonspeaking child from a family of late speakers. However, all children who are not deaf should understand speech by 15 months. Those who do not need and deserve special consideration. But we are getting a bit ahead of ourselves. The child still has an important last stage to go through before he or she becomes a full-fledged multiple-word producer. We should be mindful that even though the child may be saying a few single words, labeling people, things, and perhaps a few events, he or she is likely to continue echoic speech. Frequently, if only for the fun of it, the child will indulge in babbling and lalling.

The maintenance of echoic "responses" (echolalia) is a feature of the pseudospeech production of many autistic children. However, as I will go into later (Chapter 9), modified or mitigated echolalia may be used for communicative purposes and so is different from infant echolalia.

ANTICIPATORY LANGUAGE: DEMANDS AND COMMANDS

By 18 months, our typical child, no longer an infant or even a baby, really arrives at the magic of language. Now the child commands *mama* or *dada* or *milk* or *doddy* in order to get what he or she wants. The child is not naming, but is giving orders! And as these orders are obeyed, the child begins to appreciate how wonderful and how potent he or she can be as a speaker. We refer to this stage as *anticipatory language*, in which the child tries to influence future events. It is true speech.

Anticipatory language is indeed true speech! There are some children, mostly among the severely mentally retarded, who may reach the *labeling* or *naming* stage but fail to progress beyond it. But when the child uses language to bring about an event, he or she changes the situation, rather than just naming or identifying it. The child also reveals that some thinking has gone on. We may assume that on the basis of a rudimentary inner language system, by talking to himself or herself, the child has rehearsed possible things to say. After the rehearsal, the child decides to speak and await results. If the results are what the child expected, the specific effort and mode of behavior are both reinforced. If calling *mama* brings mother, and if she is what the child wanted and still wants, then speaking is worth the effort. If announcing *doddy* brings dolly or doggy faster than "I'll grunt and you guess," then the child has a pay-off for this new ability. So, of course, has the related adult.

Children reveal highly individual styles in their first pronouncements. A boy, who had just recently learned that he could stand on his own, literally bellowed his command, "Ball!" By this he meant, "I don't see my ball. I want it. You get it and give it to me." That's a lot to say with a single word. When his command was obeyed, he threw the ball out of his playpen and again yelled, "Ball!" This time it meant, "We're playing a game. You give me the ball, and I'll throw it away." This, we may detect, is a variety of the game we play with a trained dog. But the roles of thrower and fetcher are not altogether the same.

A friend's granddaughter revealed another style. She seemed very ladylike in asking for *doddy*. When her mother gave her the dolly, she smiled approvingly, looked down at her companion, again said "doddy," turned on her side, and closed her eyes for her nap. Within a week she said "doddy sleep." This may have meant, "Give me my dolly and we'll both take a nap," or "Give me my dolly, it's time for my nap. You're dismissed." We never found out which of the two meanings was correct. By the time the child was old enough and had language enough to tell, she had forgotten.

So it is with much of what the child intends by early pronouncements. We can only guess at meanings according to the circumstances. If the child behaves as if satisfied, we can assume that the meaning we guessed at was correct. At least, it was acceptable and satisfactory to the child. By our own behavior, by our guesses, we reinforce the meaning or meanings our children develop for the words they produce. And as we have observed, a single word may have multiple meanings.

With this magical power comes a new responsibility. Once a child shows us that he or she can speak, we expect the child to speak. Sometimes this is more than the child bargained for, but he or she learns soon enough that only within limits can one have one's own way. The guessing game holds only for what the child has not yet put into words. But once a child expresses wishes and feelings, he or she is held responsible for more of the same. It is up to the parents to make "more of the same" worthwhile. If not, the child may regress to earlier stages when, though he or she may not have gotten things as quickly, life may have been a bit easier and perhaps even a bit better.

All the early stages in speech development, from early crying to the imperious stage of anticipatory speech, are summarized in Table 2.2. It also shows what physical skills the baby can be expected to have at each stage of speech development.

HELPING THE CHILD
OFF TO A GOOD START

It is the rare and truly exceptional child who needs to be *taught* to talk. Almost all children acquire language the same way that song birds "learn" to sing or so-called talking birds "learn" to imitate human speakers. The method is simply to expose the child to a speaker or speakers with whom

Table 2.2. Milestones from Birth to 18 Months

Approximate Age	Baby Says	Baby Responds
Birth–4 weeks	Cries whenever uncomfortable, with no apparent difference in crying because of the specific cause.	Cries, eats, or sleeps. Most physical (motor) behavior involves the entire body. Flailing movements of arms and legs when crying.
4–16 weeks	Coos and makes "laughing" noises. Vocal play produces vowels and some consonant sounds involving tongue and lip activity. May engage in vocal "dialogue" with mother.	Shows awareness and need for human sounds; turns head in the direction of the source of the sound. Usually is able to support head when lying "face down." By end of this period, is likely to discover and inspect own hand.
20–24 weeks	Vocalizes when comfortable. Vowellike cooing and considerable babbling, with consonants modifying the identifiable vowels. Makes some nasal sounds (m, n) and some lip sounds, including lip vibrations suggesting a "Bronx cheer."	Sits up with support. Arm and leg movements better controlled. May be able to pick up a cube.
6–7 months	Babbling now includes self-imitation (lalling). Many of the sound productions resemble one-syllable utterances that may include ma, da, di, and do.	Sits without props, using hands if necessary for support. Increased deftness in picking up objects. Can reach with either hand. Smiles at own image.
8–9 months	Considerable self-imitative sound play. Is also likely to imitate (echo) syllables, words, and intonation patterns of older speakers.	Can stand up, holding onto an object for support. Can grasp a small object with thumb in position. Can pull a string to get an object.
10–11 months	Repeats the words of others with increased proficiency. Responds appropriately to many word cues for familiar things and "happenings." The precocious child may have several words in his (more likely her) vocabulary.	Indicates understanding of many verbal directions by appropriate behavior. Cooperates in games. Can pull himself up to a standing position. May take a side step while holding onto a fixed object.
12 months	Still likely to imitate the speech of others, but so proficiently that he sounds as if he has quite a lot to say. First labeling (identification) words for most children.	May stand without support. May walk if held by one hand. Some children may take first steps alone. Most will "walk" on hands and feet.

(continued)

Table 2.2. (*Continued*)

Approximate Age	Baby Says	Baby Responds
By 18 months	Increases word inventory, possibly from 3 to 50 words. Vocalizations reveal intonational (melody) pattern of adult speakers. May begin to use two-word utterances.	Walks without support. Runs. Can manage cubes well enough to build a two-block tower. May begin to show hand preference. Can throw a ball and turn pages of a book.

he or she can identify. Then the child will unconsciously imitate the speech heard. The imitation is, of course, not complete. The child selects from all sounds heard only those that he or she can produce. The result is infant speech. Later, in ways that are still mysterious, the magic of infant speech gives way to the supermagic of grown-up speech. Sounds become sharpened and words more readily identifiable. The child also learns the way we string words together to make statements and ask questions. This last process is called *grammar* or *syntax*.

What kind of environment encourages a child to speak? Most simply stated, one in which there is talking, but it is not a Tower of Babel. The talking should suggest pleasure or comfort, rather than anger or discomfort. When you, a parent, or other caretaker is talking directly to a baby, use short simple statements. Punctuate the flow of talk with short pauses. The pauses should be frequent and well spaced, so that the child is not overwhelmed by the quantity of sounds to which he or she is directly exposed.

The child's parents and other people who care for the child should speak as they feed, burp, change the child's linen, or whatever. They should describe what they are doing in single words or short phrases. Thus *dolly* or *milk* or *cookie* may be starters. Phrases such as *baby's doll* or *milk-baby* or *baby-cookie* may follow. If you have an urge to make a complete statement, then "Here's your dolly," or "Up we go," are fine. But avoid long and involved observations such as "Baby wants her dolly now, doesn't she?" Such a half statement, half question is too complicated for a young child to manage.

If parents and caretakers follow these suggestions—and for most parents this approach is easy and natural—then there is little else we need to be concerned about. However, because some parents may still be concerned, I will make a few additional observations.

- I emphasize that, in acquiring language, each child develops at his or her own rate. A slower than "average" rate of language acquisition does not mean that the child is retarded. (The exceptions, as indicated earlier, are only for children who do not comprehend speech, children who cannot hear, children who in other ways indicate that they are severely mentally retarded, and the autistic.)

- Language acquisition is related to some factors over which the child has no control. Girls tend to start earlier than boys and are likely to progress faster than boys up to about 3 years of age. First children, probably because they receive more complete attention from their parents than second or third children, usually progress faster than their younger sisters or brothers. However, if the age difference between children is 5 years or more, the later child is essentially like another first child.
- An important point: Available parents and other caretakers who are attentive and loving are much more helpful than those who are available but anxious.
- The child will have little use for language unless associated with pleasure and "payoff."
- Children enjoy making sounds for the fun of it, even after they can say a few words. Do nothing to discourage such sounds-for-the-fun-of-it games. You might even join in, if doing so doesn't put a stop to the game.
- Children must hear good speech if they are to become proficient speakers. Speak a bit more slowly than you would to older children or adults. Speak concisely. When you finish a statement, pause for a second or two before you make another. Don't interrupt a child's turn-taking.

Parents, grandparents, and caretakers in general should always remember that each child is unique. No infant has a contract or obligation to perform as average children are supposed to perform. The notion of average is a statistic based on a range of findings. Children, who are unaware of averages and norms, may be ahead of schedule in some ways (even in many ways) and behind in others. Some children talk before they walk (mine did) and others walk before they talk. Some children add to the comprehension and speaking vocabularies in increments that are almost regular and predictable. Other children progress by spurts and tantalizing plateaus. Most plateaus, however, are periods when the child is consolidating previous gains. A great deal is going on inside that is not readily apparent in the child's outward speech and behavior.

In deciding how well their child's speech is developing, parents would be wise to assume a month's leeway up to a year of age, and perhaps 2 months leeway from then to 1½ years of age. If the parents know that children on either side of the family are slow to talk or slow to walk, that information rather than the milestones in Table 2.2 should form the basis for their expectations. Illness delays development and sometimes results in a temporary setback. Parents should take this into account.

At best, the milestones tell us about "average" children born after a full-term healthy pregnancy. The premature child is likely to be a slow-developing child. This is especially so for the child who is born in the seventh month of pregnancy (or sooner) and who weighs less than 5 pounds. Although we can provide no formula and no schedule for the speech and motor development of premature children, we can provide a rough guide. Allow at least 2 months of postbirth time for each month of prematurity. The best guides can only be provided by a pediatrician, who will assess the child's reflexes and developmental skills. Even then, projections (still only approximate) for the child's future development need to be based on periodic reassessments.

Evaluation Instruments

There are probably 50 or more tests and evaluation procedures for approximating the language development of young children. Most, however, are not prognostic instruments that consider early infant responses to sounds (noises, both animal and human). Nor do they include the earliest vocalizations of infants. Exceptions to this observation include the Utah Test of Language Development (Mecham, Jex, & Jones, 1967) and the Receptive-Expressive Emergent Language Scale (Bzock & League, 1971). Almost all of the tests and procedures are a bit weak in validity and reliability.

A recently published instrument, the Early Language Milestone Scale (The ELM Scale) (Coplon, 1983), provides a quick screening–evaluation approach for children and gives promise for meeting the criticisms directed at most of the other published tests. The ELM Scale (see Figure 2.6) is intended for use by physicians and other professionals who have a primary concern for the welfare of infants and young children. The target populations include infants from birth to 36 months and older, developmentally delayed children who, on observation, are presumed to have less than a 36-month level of language ability. Administration time is about 3 minutes.

Coplon's premise for the ELM Scale is that mapping a baby's language development provides a reasonable means for assessing the integrity of the various neural subsystems involved in the acquisition (comprehension and production) of language. Coplon, a pediatrician, argues that "language development is a far more reliable indicator of overall developmental integrity than gross motor milestones, which are usually within normal limits in the hearing impaired or mentally retarded child."

Through the child's history, direct tests, and incidental observations, the ELM Scale evaluates the visual and auditory receptive and expressive functions of language. Forms have specific notations of items to be eval-

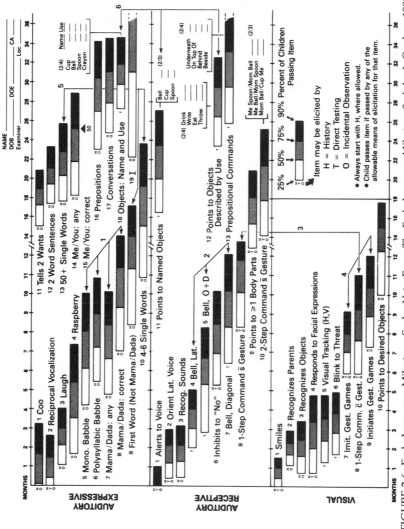

FIGURE 2.6. Early Language Milestone Scale. *Note.* From *The Early Language Milestone Scale* by J. Coplon, 1983, Tulsa, OK: Modern Education Corporation. Copyright 1983 by the Modern Education Corporation. Used with permission.

27

uated and based on Coplon's data, percentile values may be noted that correspond to the age of emergence for each item. The manual for the ELM Scale includes specific instructions for eliciting responses and filling out forms for evaluations.

Coplon (1983) alerts us that ''although the pattern of item failure on the ELM Scale may suggest a specific developmental diagnosis, the ELM Scale is intended as a screening instrument, *not* a definitive diagnostic tool. Children who fail the ELM Scale should undergo formal developmental testing, including at a minimum both audiological and psychological or speech–language evaluation'' (p. 2).

Chapter 3

First Sentences: The Language of Anticipation and Control

Next to talking and walking, most parents express the concern, "When do we start toilet training our baby?" A pediatrician friend has a standard answer for this query: "When your child puts two words together." Once, we overheard a parent ask, "Why then? How is putting two words together related to toilet training?" We also overheard his answer, "Because before then is too soon. The right time is when Bobby puts two words together."

I pondered this question for some years, about my own children, and later, my grandchildren, and in the interests of many other children. The pediatrician was usually right, but why? Now I believe I know the answer. Interestingly, the answer is directly related to the child's stage in language development. This, in turn, is related to the *child's general ability to anticipate events*.

THE LANGUAGE OF ANTICIPATION

In Chapter 2, we left the child using language as commands. Joannie and Johnny, in addition to labeling, were using words to get people to do their bidding. Parents may wonder why so often their 15- to 18-month-old child says "toity" or "wuh" (for wet) at first only after the deed is done. This, we may recognize, is just another instance of the child's naming ability. Only when the children are able to anticipate *what is about to happen*, when they can both cue and control themselves, can they announce what needs to be done before it is too late. When the child makes a noise, whether it is a grunt or sounds like a word, that serves as a signal of what is about to happen, the child also signals that he or she is ready to be toilet trained. In effect, the child is now demonstrating the ability to associate an inner

29

feeling with a consequence, and a consequence with a word. Every care-taker knows that just because this can be done is no assurance that it will be done, at least not regularly. On occasion, the child may be too busy with other matters to pay attention to these inner biological happenings. The child may simply not be aware of what is going on or, if aware, may not seem to care. So accidents do and will happen. However, if the rewards are worth the control, accidents become rare, and toilet training is achieved. Parents may take pride in knowing that this control, like speech, is peculiar to human beings.

By the time a Johnny or Joannie, or Adam or Eve, can say "Baby-toity" or Baby-wuh (wet)" in order to stay clean or dry, he or she usually has a vocabulary of about 50 recognizable words. In addition, the child may have 3–5 two-word "sentences," and at the same time, is learning to say a great deal with single words. Each word may be used not only to label but to command. A one-word command may have several meanings. In effect, this makes the single word the equivalent of several full statements. For example, *cup* may simply mean "this thing is called a cup" or possibly "I see that we have a new cup," or "come now, it's time to fill the cup." How does a parent know which meaning is intended? Only by observ-ing the child's actions and accompanying gestures.

But it is just as important for the parent to listen to the vocal inflection. Simple naming is likely to be done with a fairly flat vocal inflection, like

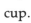
cup.

A command to "fill the cup" will have a more imperious downward in-flection:

cup.

If the child thinks it may be a cup but you never can tell, the inflection is likely to be rising:

cup.

This is the way speakers of English use voice inflections to make a varie-ty of statements and to ask questions that can ordinarily be answered by a yes or no.

COMBINING WORDS
INTO SENTENCES

Some children make the most out of these single-word sentences before they combine two or more words into new constructions. By 24 months most children have begun to use two-word sentences and some have progressed to three words. If a youngster at this age has not yet reached this stage but is using single words to indicate a variety of meanings, there is no cause for concern. Suppose, however, that the youngster was a late starter who didn't begin to use recognizable words until 18 months of age. In that case, allow some added time for catching up. A late starter may not begin to use two-word combinations until 30 months of age.

At all times *what is important to notice is whether there is progress in some direction relative to language comprehension or production.* Does the child understand more of what he or she hears? Is the child speaking more of the time, either using more words or suggesting more meanings for the words used? To know for sure, parents need to keep notes and records. They should chart the course of language development over periods of weeks and months rather than days. Somehow, after long enough intervals of time, almost all children achieve approximately the same goal. They understand what you say and, in turn, speak so that you understand them. But each child gets there by a unique route.

The production of *two-word combinations* marks a new and important stage in the child's language development. For most children, this stage usually begins when the child has a vocabulary of at least 50 single-word sentences. A child may achieve this level of development as early as 18 months of age or as late as 30 to 36 months of age. Most children are likely to use two-word combinations by 24 months.

The child uses two-word combinations, just as earlier he or she used single words, for a variety of meanings. For example, *mommy-shoe* may mean: "Please, mommy, put on my shoes" or "Mommy is putting on my shoes" or "Mommy, put on your shoes so that we can get going." The combination *baby-milk* may mean: "I want milk" or "You are about to give me milk" or "I want more milk."

CREATIVE LANGUAGE AND THE USE OF SYNTAX

Somtimes during the two-word-combination stage, most children will begin to say things they have *not* been specifically "taught." For example, a child who has been "taught" to say "Baby up" may, *on his own,* say "Daddy up" or "Mommy up."

When children do this they are demonstrating that they learn more than their caretakers "teach" them. What parents or caretakers teach a child, or think they have taught, serves as a model. The child uses this model to try out new word combinations. He or she may even reverse the order of the words. Instead of saying "Baby up," the child may try out "Up baby" and "Up dolly" and "Up ball." Now the child has become a *creative speaker* and is making it clear not only that he or she understands you but also that this understanding can be generalized. In a very real sense, the child is a generator of new constructions based on models of "old" constructions. Now all that is left in order to become expert in the language game is to build up a vocabulary and learn more about how grown-ups string words together and speak in their harried and breathless way.

The period between 18 and 36 months is one of rapid growth in all aspects of language. At 18 months, a child may have a speaking vocabulary of about 50 words. By 36 months this vocabulary may increase to 1000 words or more. Figure 3.1 shows the unusually rapid growth of vocabulary between the ages of 2 and 3. Of course, vocabulary growth never ends. We continue to learn new words and new meanings of words until we are no longer capable of learning.

LANGUAGE MILESTONES FROM AGES TWO TO FOUR

By the age of 2, most children have achieved the following:

- They understand hundreds of words and many thousands of sentences that include the words they know.
- They begin to use new combinations, based on models or representative sentences that others use. So, now the child who has been "trained" or "taught" the construction, "Where is the dolly?" knows where to look or that he should start looking when he hears, "Where is the doggy?" Similarly, the child who has as his model "Baby-shoe" may himself begin to say "Baby-sock" or "Baby-hat." Children who can do this are creative listeners and creative talkers. They are able to understand things they never heard before and say things they never tried before *with full anticipation of being understood*.

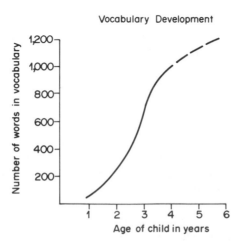

FIGURE 3.1. Vocabulary development.

- The child begins to string words together—that is, to use syntax—in the manner of the grown-up speakers in the immediate environment. By 4 years of age, most children are fairly proficient in the use of syntax. By age 5, all but a small percentage of children are almost as proficient as most of the adults in their homes.

Anticipation, Regulation, and Control

Although Table 3.1 will bring us up to age 4, let's concentrate on the highly significant accomplishments in the use of language by most 2 year olds. At this age, children who have begun to put words together in sentences indicate that they are serious communicators. In their statements, and later in their questions, these 2 year olds expect something to happen as a consequence of what they say and how they say it. If their expectations are not met, we may be treated to demonstrations of what is meant by the *terrible twos*. At this age, we may observe *self-awareness* and *anticipatory awareness*—their anticipations according to their standards of how others are supposed to relate and behave toward them *when they speak*!

Halliday (1975) classifies the communicative efforts of 2 year olds into three broad categories: interaction, regulation, and personal control. These communicative categories serve seven functions:

1. Instrumental—language used to satisfy specific material needs: "I (me) want kitty," "I want cookie," "I want (something material)."
2. Regulatory—language to exert control or direct the behavior of another person: "Daddy come," "Mommy up."
3. Interactional (social gesture)—language used to establish or maintain contact with an important other person; for example, "Please, mommy," "Hi, gamma."
4. Heuristic—language used to investigate or explore the environment; "There doggy," "What that?"
5. Personal—language to announce and express individuality, to speak of oneself; for example, "I (me) girl," "I (me) jump," "I pretty."
6. Imaginative—language used in make-believe play or to create a pretend world; for example, "I'm a doggy," "I'm a mommy," or even, if the need arises, "Me baby."
7. Informative—in contrast to the heuristic, language employed to provide information, real or imaginary, to someone who is elected to have it. This use of language may overlap the factual; for example, "I'm a big bear" is both imaginative and informative, whereas "Puffy is my kitty" may be factual.

It is obvious that some of the functions of language overlap. For example, "I'm a big bear" may inform a listener of her expected role in a game in which the child will act out an announced role. "I jump" also serves to regulate the child's behavior.

Proficiency in Syntax:
The Grammar of Adult Language

By the age of 3 or 4, the child's ability to combine words into sentences or other meaningful combinations—that is, to use syntax—closely resembles that of the key adults in his or her special environment. The child's growth in the use of syntax and in pronouncing words clearly parallels a very rapid growth in vocabulary. Except for voice, which happily remains childish, and some "infantile" pronunciations, the child has progressed a long way toward speaking the way adults do.

Learning syntax is a tremendous accomplishment. Yet the child isn't at all aware of how difficult an achievement it is—for children beyond age 10 and for almost all adults who learn to understand and speak a second language. Here are some age-related "statistics." However difficult it is for adults to learn a second language, all but 3 to 5 percent of children learn to speak one or more languages by mere exposure if the exposure is before age 10. From ages 10 to 12, it is more difficult to learn a second language and sound like a native speaker. After age 12, second-language learning becomes even more difficult unless a person is completely immersed in the new language and avoids, at least for a time, the use of the first.

To go back to our 3-year-old child, who has already accomplished so much: He or she soon learns how to say things that indicate the present, the past, or the future and learns how complicated constructions become that begin with words such as *if* or *although*. The English-speaking child also learns what to do with words to indicate singular or plural and how to change verbs to make them "agree" with their subject words. Children who speak other languages may learn that subjects "agree" with predicates not only in number but also in gender. They learn an amazing number of ways to say complex things in complex ways. Bilingual children may learn two ways of saying the "same" thing in two languages. Almost always, they learn all these things without any awareness of the immensity of their achievement. The use of language, beyond anything else, is what it means to be a human being.

The milestones we have discussed should provide most parents with the information they need to answer the question "Is my child progressing normally in speech?" But parents, and other persons interested and involved in the development of the mentally retarded or deaf child, need to know more.

Without direct and specific teaching, severely mentally retarded children rarely go beyond the labeling stage in language acquisition. Moderately mentally retarded children are slow in combining words and slow in reaching the stage where they use conventional (adult) language constructions. Most, however, do get there. Perhaps when they are 7 or 8 years of age they are on a 3-year-old level of proficiency. But this is not too bad. A year or two later they may be almost as good as most 4 or 5 year olds. By this time, most aspects of grammar are under control. At least they are able to use and understand sentence constructions like those used by the adults around them.

Deaf children tend to be severely deficient in their use of conventional word constructions, but this may be a reflection of the way they are taught, or not taught. Hans G. Furth (1966), an authority on the deaf, observes, "Many persons whom we do not consider capable of complex intelligent behavior learn the language of our society better than the majority of pupils in our schools for the deaf." In his book *Thinking Without Language*, Furth offered suggestions on improving both the language and the thinking of the deaf. Fortunately, much of what he advised is now practiced, with positive and encouraging results.

The recent introduction of sign systems that incorporate syntactic features, word equivalence of signs, and conventional English word order, as well as pronouns, prepositions, articles, infinitives, and "function" words, brings signing closer to grammatically correct spoken English. Such systems include *SEE* (Anthony & Associates, 1971), *Signing Exact English (SEE 2)* (Gustason, Pfetzinger, & Aswolkow, 1972) and *Signed English* (Bornstein, Hamilton, Sauliner, & Roy, 1975).

From our previous discussion and from Table 3.1 it should be apparent that, for most children, the second birthday marks the start of a dramatic age. It is not only the beginning period of great physical achievement, one when the child develops physical skills and controls, but also a period in which we see evidence of rapid intellectual growth. Baby talk begins to give way to more grown-up pronunciations. Within a few months, the child may increase his or her speaking vocabulary from 50 words to several hundred. (Note that we are no longer referring to the subject of this book as a *baby* but as a *child*.) Within a year, the youngster's vocabulary may exceed 1000 words. At age 3, the child can speak his or her mind, make intentions clear, and understand an adult's intention, sometimes despite the words the adult may use.

By age 4, except possibly for the sounds *s*, *th*, *l*, and *r*, the child is proficient in controlling the sounds of the language. The child's vocabulary continues to grow rapidly, although not at the same rate it did between ages 2 and 4. He or she speaks with the syntax of the adults in the surrounding environment. Yet somehow, the child can speak not only for himself or herself but as a unique self in an individual rhetorical style.

Table 3.1. A Child's Milestones from Two to Four Years

Approximate Age	Comprehension and Language	Capability
24 months	Understands hundreds of words and sentences. Has a speaking vocabulary of 50 or more words. May begin to use two-word combinations.	Walks with relative ease. Can walk up or down stairs, usually planting both feet on each step before going to next step.
30 months	The child's vocabulary growth is proportionately greater than at any other period. Many, perhaps most, of the child's sentences are grammatically like those of the adults in his or her life. Understands most of what is said if it is within his or her experience. Articulation (pronunciation) may include some infant sounds, such as *w* for *r*, but almost all of what is said is understood by well-intentioned listeners.	Can jump and stand on one foot. Has good hand and finger coordination. Can build a tower with as many as six blocks.
36 months	Speaking vocabulary may exceed 1000 words. Syntax almost completely "grown up." Can say what he or she thinks and make intentions clear. Except for voice, the child speaks much as the older members of the community do.	Runs proficiently. Can walk stairs by alternating feet. Hand preference is usually established.
48 months	Except possibly for some difficulty with *s, th, l,* and *r,* the child's articulation (sound production) is under good control. Grammatically, the child has acquired almost as much as he or she is likely to acquire. Yet, somehow, the child still manages to have a personal style, employing favorite words and individual ways of turning a phrase (in an individual "rhetorical" style).	Can hop on one foot, usually the right one unless left-handed. Can throw a ball in the direction of an intended receiver. Can catch a ball in arms and occasionally with both hands. Can walk on a line. Is able to ride a tricycle and perhaps a small bicycle.

Again, we should be mindful that these milestones are only approximate guides to accomplishment. Not all children are equally skillful in their physical development. Some are slow in developing their skills, but catch up within 6 months or a year to "normal" or "average" expectation. What I said of physical skills also holds for speech acquisition. Do not be rigid in your interpretation of the information in the tables. The information is there only to supply approximate guides. If the child deviates too much from the guidelines—say 6 months or more—this should be of concern to the pediatrician, family physician or other professional consultant. The professional consulted should be able to answer the parent's questions or refer the parent to another professional person who can. In any event, parents do have a right to ask and a right to know!

QUESTIONS AND COGNITIVE DEVELOPMENT

Why Do Children Ask Questions?

What purposes do questions serve? Why, once they get started, do most children ask so many questions? A general answer is that children ask questions because, through the answers they receive, they can get more and learn more than they could if they didn't ask questions. At first, they want to obtain things and information about things. Later, children use questions to get information to satisfy their intellectual curiosity as well.

When children are infants, parents anticipate most of their needs. As children's minds mature, they begin to have needs that, fortunately, cannot be readily anticipated. These needs go beyond physical comfort and security. They need to know for the sake of knowing! First questions may, however, be deceiving. When the child asks "Doddy (dolly)?" or "What dat (that)?" he or she is probably trying to obtain something, rather than learn something. First questions may simply indicate that the child has discovered a new tool or technique to serve an old purpose. Thus, first questions are usually new ways with words that permit children to satisfy their needs. Later, the same device and the very same words may be used to gain information related both to earlier needs and to new ones.

Children's questions reveal that something is going on in their minds that can be satisfied only with the help of others. Presumably, these others are either more skillful, or have longer reaches or particular possessions that interest children. So children put other persons to work for them. In doing so, they become socialized. They use questions, even those used for obtaining physical things, to involve the persons around them in some kind of social cooperation. Through questions, inexperienced children make use of the experience, abilities, and knowledge of adults.

First Questions and Their Cognitive Significance

Eighteen-month-old Johnny asks "Cookie?" and indicates that he wants somebody to give him a little cake. The inflection of his voice, if Johnny is an English-speaking child, will follow this contour:

cookie.

In asking for his goodie with a single word and an upward inflection, Johnny expects, or at least hopes, that the answer will be yes. Further, he expects that appropriate action will accompany or follow the verbal response. The answer might be no, of course, but it is unlikely that a wise Johnny will ask for something that might be denied. If Johnny is not allowed to have the cookie, he may resort to an old and usually successful mode of behavior—and achieve by crying what he failed to obtain by talking.

At 18 months, the child is likely to ask questions only about things in sight, things heard, or at least things he or she can touch. The typical 18-month-old child is still pretty much tied to the here and now, to responding and dealing with matters that are part of the child's immediate experience. These experiences, literally, are ones that the child can touch, smell, and see. So the question "Cookie?" is likely to occur only when a cookie is present and in view but not in the child's reach. At a later stage in cognitive development the child may use the same single-word form to ask questions about matters not in sight, to get answers to little puzzling thoughts such as "Later?" or "Now?"

At 18 months, most children reach a two- to three-word language stage, at which they begin to combine words in statements such as "Tom ball," "John cookie," and "Kitty eat." Some of the children progress rapidly from two-word statements to longer ones, such as "Ride in wagon," or even "I (or "me") ride in wagon." We may also hear children's observations about what other children or grown-ups are doing, such as "Boy throwing ball" and "Man riding bike."

About the time when children begin to produce two- and three-word statements, they also ask their first questions that begin with interrogative (question) words. The first of these interrogative words is likely to be *where* or *what*. Usually, but by no means invariably, the future order of development for interrogative words is *who, why, how,* and *when.* Together, despite the spelling of *how*, sentences that start with interrogative words are called *wh* questions.

Except for the onset of talking, there is no better indicator that all is going well in the mental development of the child than his or her ability to understand and ask questions. Through questions, especially those that go beyond yes and no for answers, children reveal that their minds have the capacity to deal with matters that are not physically present. With the *wh* questions (where, who, what, why, how, and when) the child's mind can roam and range through time and space.

Now the child can talk and think about what happened during some yesterday, however vague that yesterday may be. The child can talk and speculate about tomorrow. Questions and questioning that began as devices for getting things done soon advance to devices for exercising imagination and testing thinking. These uses of questions should assure parents that all is going well with the child.

Different Kinds of Yes/No Questions

The earliest questions that children ask are usually designed to bring a yes or no answer—hopefully, a yes. As they grow, children discover several different ways of phrasing these yes/no questions.

Typically, in early stages, the word order of a question takes the form of a statement: "Cookie?" or "Mommy cookie?" Later, the question may be elaborated to "May I have a cookie?" The rising vocal inflection at the end of the "statement" as well as the overall structure of the utterance indicates that this is in fact a question.

The question "Dolly?" may be a polite command. The child knows that, although he or she is asking a question, *you* know that you are expected to comply as if it were a request, "Please hand me my dolly." This kind of question may be a forerunner of the adult question, "Would it trouble you to close the door?" If the answer is "No trouble at all," without any move to close the door, then the listener either didn't understand the first speaker's intention or preferred to pretend that he didn't understand it.

"Is dolly sleeping?" is a second form of the yes/no question. Now the child has learned that questions can be asked by changing the order of the words from a statement structure, as in "Dolly is sleeping" to one that begins with the verb. No matter what inflection the child uses, this form of question requires a response from a listener.

A third way to ask a yes/no question is to present the order of the words as a statement and then to tag on a *huh* or the equivalent. So we may have "The boy (is) running, huh?" The *huh* is a rough equivalent of the adult forms, *Right?* or *Yes?* or *No?* or *Isn't it?* or *Can't I?* By age 5, most children can understand as well as produce such questions.

As children learn the variety of ways to get a yes or no answer, they use the rising inflectional form alone much less often. But, as most adults know, children do not abandon this first way of asking questions. They simply acquire other ways which they employ according to circumstances, their needs, and their developing styles. Thus a 6-year-old's request for a piece of candy may take several forms:

- To a friend, also age 6: "Got one for me, huh?"
- To an adult, other than a parent: "Please, may I have a piece of candy?"
- To a parent, if the relationship is informal and cordial: "Could I have a piece of candy?" or just "Candy?"

(What would the relationship be if a 6-year-old asks a parent, "Please, I would like a candy?")

Interrogative Word Questions:
Wh- and How

Where. "*Where* boy run?" "*Where* that?" "*Where* mommy going?" These are examples of early *where* questions. In 2 or 3 months, the child may ask the same question in a more complete grammatical form, such as "Where is the boy running?" or "Where is that?" or even "Where is daddy going?" The child expects that the answer will be a location word or phrase. So, whether it is "Where boy run?" or "Where is the boy running?" an answer such as "To his house" or "To the store" is appropriate.

A little later in the child's career, a location word answer may not be enough. The child may continue the questioning by asking "Why?" We will not pretend to have an adequate answer to *why* questions, which we discuss again a little later. Caretakers will have to figure out these answers according to their own intellectual resources. Children who are acquisitive need to be inquisitive (that is, children who are acquiring language need to ask questions) and older persons are supposed to fall in line by providing answers. *What* and *where* questions are usually easy to answer. *Why* questions are a challenge to intellect, imagination, and endurance. For whatever comfort it may provide to caretakers, the number of questions that begin with *why* increases with the child's age, intellectual development, and language proficiency.

Who. *Who*, the child somehow learns, is reserved for persons and respected animals. He or she may begin to use *who* even before adult forms of the question are mastered. So we may get "Who that?" or, more likely, "Who dat?" several months before "Who is that?" The question form *who* may be used by the child to engage a parent in conversation. For example, a child may point to a girl or a boy in a picture and ask the parent "Who is throwing ball?" or to a baby and ask "Who is sleeping?" If the parent answers appropriately, the child may keep the game going of *I point and ask and you tell.* Lucky parents usually have a turn to ask questions and to approve of their child's answers.

Later *who* questions may take the more adult form of "Who is eating the candy?" or "Who is driving the car?" or "Who is the girl helping?"*

---

*The subtitle distinction between *who* and *whom* (the subject word and the object word in formal "old fashioned" grammar) is likely to escape even the most inquisitive child for many years. Early use is almost limited to *who* as the subject or object in the sentence.

What. *What* questions come early in the child's career as a speaker. Most children ask "What dat (that)?" shortly after they begin to put two words together in a single utterance. "What dat?" may be a real question or a pseudoquestion. In fact, *what* is likely to be used simply to engage an adult in conversation before it is used to obtain information. Even then it is interesting to note that the child is asking for a name and so perhaps may be going through a second naming stage. This time, however, the child is getting someone else to supply the names of things.

As the child develops a sense of grammar, the form of the *what* questions is likely to be close to that of an adult's. Then we may hear "What is that?" and "What is mommy carrying?" The child is still asking that something be named. Soon, however, the child may ask that events and actions be named, as in "What boy do?" and, later, the adult form, "What is the boy doing?" and "What is the girl (or mommy or daddy) reading?" Often, we suspect, children ask *what* questions to make sure of certain names and information rather than to obtain new names or new information. The parent should play along with the child in this "game," even when the parent knows that the child knows and the child knows that the parent knows. Children as well as adults have a right to ask rhetorical and pretend questions, as well as genuine information-seeking questions.

What if questions are a long leap in mental development from the *what* questions, even though the child advances to them rather soon after framing the first *what* questions. When the child asks questions like "What *if* it rains?" or "What *if* daddy comes late?" the parent knows that the child can now deal with future and uncertain events, with abstractions. *What if* questions keep parents sharp in their thinking and in their intellectual resources—a very good state of affairs for all members of a family.

Why. As most parents of 2-year-olds have learned, there is no limit to the number of situations about which children ask *why*. Children, if they are a bit on the precocious side, begin to ask about the *why* of matters as early as 18 months. Some of the *why* questions are a bit perplexing to adults because the answers lie within the child's own experience. Here is an actual dialogue between a mother and a 20-month-old child:

> *Child*: Why me pill [spill] milk?
> *Mother*: You were not looking.
> *Child*: Why not me not looking?

We suspect that if there was an answer to this child's question, only the child could provide it. However, it is likely that the child was engaging in social dialogue, perhaps to divert the mother's attention from the minor but recurrent catastrophe of milk spilling.

More conventional but not necessarily easier *why* questions may be asked about anything that comes to a child's attention.

- "Why is girl riding?"
- "Why is baby sleeping?"
- "Why is mommy sitting?" (or reading, or cooking, or whatever)

Later, *why* questions are likely to be asked in adult grammatical form: "Why is the boy laughing?" or "Why are the birds flying?" When the child is about 4, we may expect to be asked *why* questions that call for explanations rather than a mere statement of information. "Why are the birds flying" is such a question. "Why did the bird die?" or "Why does the wind blow?" call for answers that involve cause and effect. Such questions reveal that the child's thinking is no longer tied to immediate physical needs or situations. They reveal intellectual curiosity about natural phenomena. They reveal intellectual growth that should be highly pleasing to parents.

How. *How* questions occur relatively late in the child's development as a question-asker. Early *how* questions suggest that although using *how*, the child really *intends* to ask *why*. "How is the boy crying?" and "How is the boy eating?" represent first attempts at the use of *how*, but probably really mean *why*. Later *how* questions, when children are in their third and fourth years, are more likely to mean *how* in the adult sense. Then we may hear, "How does a bird (or an airplane) fly?" or "How are clouds made?" or, rarely, "How can I help you, mommy?"

At 4 or 5 years of age, children may ask "How do flowers grow?" or "How is snow made?" We assume that parents of children who are curious enough and bright enough to ask such questions are themselves bright enough to provide satisfactory answers.

When. *When* questions also begin relatively late in the child's career as a questioner. Two- and three-year-old children, unless they are precocious intellectually and in language development, ask few *when* questions. Occasionally, we may hear *when* used for *what* or *why* as in "When is the boy touching?" and "When is the boy laughing?"

Usually, by the time children acquire *when* in their inventory of question words, they are likely to use grown-up grammar. "When is Mary's party?" or "When is Bobby's birthday?" are typical examples. However, we also have the example of "When is it winter?" asked by a 2½ year old. The question "When will it work, dad?" was asked by a 4-year-old boy who was watching his father make adjustments to the family television set.

Children Who Ask Few Questions

Some children are slow to begin to ask questions, and continue to ask relatively few questions after they have begun. My investigations indicate that there are three groups of children like this.

The first group consists of children who are either ignored or rejected. The rejection may take the form of a thoughtless and unreasonable "No," or a response in the form of "Don't ask so many questions." Parents who are guilty of either the unreasoned "No" or the discouraging "Don't ask . . . " might ask themselves the following:

- What does a child need to do to get yes for an answer?
- How many questions would not be too many?
- What should the child do as a substitute for asking questions? (This may be the most important question of all.)

If these questions are answered honestly, most parents will discover that they want their children to continue with the questions, and that they are willing to begin to answer.

A second group of children who ask few questions and begin to ask them rather late in their careers are those who are slow in mental development. Interestingly, however, the order of questions these children ask parallels that of normal and bright children.

A third group of children who are both slow starters and reluctant questioners, but not intellectually retarded, are ones who are severely delayed in language acquisition. This is a very special but small group of children, some of whom are brain damaged, who are very slow in speech development. Some of them may not have spoken their first words by age 4 or 5. Many of them appear to be unable to learn to speak by normal exposure to speaking adults. They need to be directly taught because of their severe limitation for learning and acquiring language by exposure.

This very special group is the subject of the book *Aphasia and Related Disorders in Children* (Eisenson, 1984a). I have studied more than 100 of these children and discovered that even at ages 9 and 10, when they have overcome most of their language delay, they still seem disinclined to ask questions. This is both surprising and perplexing because, even after they have demonstrated that they do comprehend questions of all types and on occasion can use question constructions, they are much less likely to do so, compared with younger children on the same level of language development. A possible explanation for this apparent disinclination is that the use of the interrogative implies an ability and willingness to deal with the abstract. Aphasic children, as a total population, are more concrete minded and more inclined to deal with the here and now, with objective realities, that do not ordinarily require the use of question constructions. This conjecture would particularly hold for *why*, *when*, and *how* words in *wh* questions.

Alternative Strategies to Asking Questions

Are children who ask few questions necessarily those who are or were delayed in language development? Not at all, if there is no other indication of language delay and especially if the child has effective strategies to get answers and actions without having to ask questions. My granddaughter, for reasons I was not able to discern, asked very few questions at an age when most of her peers discovered the wonder of *wh* words. Although she asked few questions, she was able to get many answers. Her strategy might be identified as positive thinking. For instance, if she wanted to visit a friend or favorite relative, she was likely to say to her parents, "Tomorrow, let's go visit David." This manner of indicating her wish often resulted in a fairly lengthy dialogue, which she expected and in which she held her own. (As a grandparent I might note that she began holding her own moments after she was born.) By age 3, sharpened and motivated by competition with her 6-year-old brother, she was not only highly proficient in language but also fully able to protect her rights and privileges through actions as well as words. At bedtime, my granddaugther collected her books and then addressed a selected, privileged relative with "It's story reading time." As an admiring but still objective observer, it was clear that this granddaughter did not resort to questions; neither did she entertain any doubt that her statement (invitation) would produce the action she expected to follow.

As with older children and adults, asking a question may frequently be a way of opening a dialogue, a social interchange with another potential speaker. The answer, whether it is a direct response to the question, indicates a willingness to continue the dialogue. Children learn this use of "questions" by observing adults play this social–verbal game.

There are many young granddaughters and grandsons who ask questions—especially *why*, *how*, and *when* questions—perhaps more often than most children. *What if* questions may occur more often than the simple *what*. For reasons that are only subjective and personal, I consider children to be on the bright side who can and do ask questions and who use alternative strategies as well for getting the answers and the actions they want. In this respect, children who frequently or occasionally use alternative strategies fulfill the two basic functions served by questions.

Initially, questions are social tools. Through asking questions, children get other persons involved in the satisfaction of their needs. At first, these needs are usually actions that cannot be accomplished alone by the questioner, because the cookie or the friend or the relative is beyond easy reach. Later, the child may seek information, or want confirmation of what he or she already knows, from an esteemed listener. Finally, children seek explanations as well as information and confirmation. They may, of course, still be making sure of their own observations and explanations. Questions and still more questions, or alternative strategies for asking questions, are expressions of maturing minds. The answers children receive are the reflections of maturing adults.

Questions in Form but Not Intent

"Why don't you close the door when you come in?" "Do you mind turning down the radio?" "How many times must I ask you to wash your hands before you eat?" These are examples of pseudoquestions that the young child is exposed to and learns do not really call for answers that inform, explain, affirm, or negate. What the child learns also is to appreciate the intended rather than the literal meaning of a message. In these instances, the message is presented in the form and disguise of a question.

When an adult asks a child "Is this a green or red ball?" the likelihood is that, unless the questioner is color blind, the purpose of the "question" is not a request for information but rather a way to determine a child's knowledge of red and green. Sometimes, it is used to teach these colors. This form of "questioning" may also be used to show off a child's knowledge to another person, who is to be impressed.

Although young children are not likely to use these pseudoquestions in self-initiated dialogues with adults, they may and do use them in play with their peers or their dolls or stuffed animals and sometimes with their live pets, who are not expected to respond.

Later Questions

Between ages 3 and 4, children are able to ask questions that include a negative word in the interrogative form. Examples are "Can't Bobby play?" "Why won't Bobby play?" "Won't we go to the park?" or "Why don't we eat now?" These are sophisticated forms of questions that reveal an ability to employ complex grammatical constructions. When children are able to ask such questions, they are also able to construct such complex sentences as "Mommy feeds the baby who is hungry" and "Mary drinks the juice because she is thirsty." They may also appreciate the subtle distinction between "Do you want to go?" and "Don't you want to go?"

In summary, children use questions or strategies to avoid possible No answers to some questions, to reveal their thinking. They also reveal that their talking is no longer restricted to the here and now. Early questions, like early statements, reflect needs for names or children's desires for getting someone to do something they cannot do for themselves. Their questions—or perhaps the process of questioning—permit a delay in action and the involvement of another person in a contemplated action. Later questions (questioning) may be used to make sure of certain information or to gather information and opinion as to the *whys, why nots,* and *hows* of what is happening in a world bounded only by the child's imagination.

Children also learn that things are not always what they seem to be, in the way adults use question constructions for a variety of purposes that are a far cry from the first questions addressed to or asked by them. What they are learning is related to the pragmatics of language usage, how to say what you need to say to enhance the likelihood that your message will be understood and you will get what you want.

Chapter 4
Articulation: Intelligible Speech

HOW INTELLIGIBLE SHOULD A CHILD'S SPEECH BE?

Articulation refers to the related, synchronized behaviors involved in modifying—molding, shaping, partially or momentarily interrupting and then releasing—the flow of breath to produce the sound-symbols of a language system. Articulation, if proficient, makes speech intelligible. If articulation is defective, intelligibility is likely to be reduced. Deficiencies in articulation account for about 75% of children's speech-communicative disorders.

Variations from proficient adult articulation do not necessarily constitute defects in childhood. Our expectations of preschool age children should be different and more liberal than those we may have for older children and adults. We can sum up normal expectations by recalling—as I have often done for parents—the biblical observation from *Corinthians*: "When I was a child, I spoke as a child, I understood as a child, I thought as a child; but when I became a man, I put away childish things."

A child is entitled to have childish, even infantile, speech. Not until children are 7 or 8 years of age should we expect most of them to put aside childish speech, if not childish thoughts. Then, except for vocal pitch range and voice quality, they do in fact begin to speak like adults. That is, their spoken communications should be intelligible and their articulation adult in proficiency.

Another answer to "How distinct should a child's speech be?" is "Distinct enough so that the child's messages are intelligible." Intelligibility—how easily a message can be understood—depends on many things, on the listener as well as the speaker. Fathers often have a harder time understanding (decoding) the speech of their children than mothers. Older children frequently do much better than either parent. In fact, in some families, big brothers and sisters are the official interpreters for the household.

Speech should become more distinct, of course, as the child grows older. Speech that is distinct enough (decodable) for a 12- to 18-month-old child is "below standard of acceptability" for a 2-year-old. What we find acceptable for a 2-year-old is in turn below what we expect for a 3-year-old.

Distinctness in speech depends on several factors.

- Articulation: Production of the sounds of a given language system
- Pronunciation: A combination of articulation and syllable stress
- Phrasing: The grouping of words
- Patterns of inflection: The intonation or contours of speech

As listeners, we do not ordinarily analyze which of these factors makes for or detracts from an intelligible message. But each factor, if it deviates too much from what we expect, can make decoding very difficult. This is especially true if the message is long or complicated and we have had little opportunity to "tune in."

THE SOUNDS OF INFANCY: EARLY ARTICULATION

Occasionally, we discover a beginning speaker, usually a girl, who somehow speaks like an adult with the first words. But most beginning speakers do just what we would expect. They speak like infants, with a very small inventory of sounds. Since infant speakers, presumably, do not have much to say and since most adults are decently tolerant, infant speech is decodable. That is, babies speak intelligibly enough to express their little messages.

If we examine their early, usually single word messages, for what infants need to say, we will have a pretty good idea of infant articulation. Children's first words are, as indicated earlier, likely to include the social gestures "hi" and "bye-bye" or their equivalents. Not surprisingly, first words also include names that can soon be used as commands for parents and other caretakers, for things they need for play or comfort (ball, dolly, peek-a-boo) and for whatever else it takes to make life comfortable. First words are also likely to include commands to initiate, maintain, or stop an action. These may be the same words used to name something or somebody but with a vocal inflection that at first may sound like a request but, if the adult does not catch on, changes to the voice of command. "No" and "more" are used with increasing frequency.

The following list is a likely first vocabulary, with spelling adjusted to suggest actual pronunciations.

- hi: greeting, often with gesture
- ba-ba: bye-bye (may also be used for baby or ball)

- dada: father or an adult male
- mama: mother or an adult woman
- daddy or gaggy: dolly or dog or stuffed animal toy
- puh-puh: papa if distinguished from dada; grandpa
- gumma: grandmother
- gubba or gumba: grandfather
- pitty: pretty
- wa-wa: water, drink
- pee-pee: peek-a-boo
- nanna: grandmother, caretaker
- nuh-nuh: no
- maw or ma or mama: more, or to continue an action, mother

This list provides us with several recurrent features of "infantile" articulation:

1. The duplication of syllables.
2. The use of sounds produced in the front of the mouth (*m, d, p, b, n*).
3. The high frequency use of breath-stopping sounds (*d, p, b, g*).
4. The use of nasally emitted sounds (*m, n*).

The sounds of the first words are for the most part consonants with one or two vowels standing for any vowel. As the child increases needs and vocabulary, the same sounds at first are likely to be used in place of others in more grown-up pronunciations. These will be considered later.

We may note that the listed likely first words are produced with only 7 consonants and 4 vowels (actually 3 vowels and 1 diphthong for the word *hi*). The vowel *a* (ä) is the most frequently used. Table 4.1 lists the sounds (phonemes) of American English. Although our spelling somehow represents them with 26 letters, we have 25 consonants, 15 vowels, and 3 stable diphthongs. Normally, by age 4 or 5, most of these sounds are under control and there should be minimum evidence of infantalisms. By age 7, articulation and pronunciation should be of adult level of proficiency. Table 4.2 indicates the expected age for sound control.

Many children get along with only 10 basic sounds—a single vowel and 9 consonants— for 6 months to a year after they say their first words. By 4 years of age, most of the sounds of the language are under good control. English-speaking children may continue to have some difficulty with the *s, l, r* and *th* sounds. By 7 or 8, even these difficulties are likely to have been overcome, and children articulate much as adults do. Some children, more likely girls than boys, reach this adultlike proficiency by the time they reach 5 years of age.

A few children, mostly those who have impaired hearing and some who for other reasons are delayed in their speech development, seem to have

Table 4.1. The Common Phonemes
(Speech Sounds) of
American English Consonants

Key Word	Most Frequent Dictionary Symbol	IPA* Symbol
1. pad	p	p
2. beet	b	b
3. tip	t	t
4. den	d	d
5. cook, came	k	k
6. gate	g	g
7. fat	f	f
8. vane	v	v
9. thin	th	θ
10. this	~~th~~	ð
11. see	s	s
12. zoo	z	z
13. shoe	sh	ʃ
14. measure	zh	ʒ
15. chip	ch	tʃ
16. jam	j	dʒ
17. me	m	m
18. no	n	n
19. ring	ng	ŋ
20. let	l	l
21. run	r	r
22. yet	y	j
23. hat	h	h
24. win	w	w
25. what	hw	ʍ or hw

*International Phonetic Alphabet

difficulty with grammar. If they do, these children may not say the final *s*, *t*, and *d* sounds because they don't understand how to form plural words or words in the past tense or how to indicate possession. These omissions are not errors of articulation.

Occasionally, we observe regressions. Even normal children sometimes slip backward in their speech proficiency. It is as if the child recalls that he still has the right to speak like a child, to lisp his *s* and *z* sounds, and to substitute a *w* for an *l* or an *r*. These substitutions are called *infantilisms*. They may indeed indicate that, for the moment at least, the child wishes to be a baby again or even that the burdens of childhood are too great. Ordinarily, these infantilisms are but a passing phase in social development. I don't recommend correcting them until the child is at least 6 or 7 years old. Even then, it may be better to deal with the cause—the reason for the child's need to be infantile—than to treat the symptom.

THE SOUNDS OF GROWING UP

Earlier, I reviewed the sounds that children are likely to use in their first 25–100 words. Although adult proficiency in sound production varies from child to child, most children achieve this level of control by age 6 or 7, perhaps more so for girls than for boys. Unless a child has a low frequency hearing loss, vowels are generally controlled by age four. In checking for proficiency, it is more important to note whether there is continued progress rather than deviation from age norms.

TONGUE TRIPPERS

English speech has many combinations or blends of sounds, such as *dr* in *drink, bl* in *blue, sp* in *spoon, fl* as in *fly,* and *st* and *sk* as in *steak* and *skip.* There are also triple-sound blends such as *sks* and *str* as in *asks* and *street.* Even at age 7, these blends may not be produced proficiently, although the

Table 4.2. The Common Phonemes of American English:
Vowels and Diphthongs

Key Word	Dictionary Symbol	IPA Symbol
1. feet	ē	i
2. sip	ĭ	ɪ
3. bake	ā	e
4. pet	ĕ	ε
5. map	ă	æ
6. ask	ă or à	æ or a according to regional or individual variations
7. palm	ä	ɑ
8. cot	ŏ or ä	ɒ or ɑ according to regional or individual variations
9. saw	ô	ɔ
10. note	ō	o or ou
11. full	o͝o	ʊ
12. toot	o͞o	u
13. puff	ŭ	ʌ
14. about	ə	ə
15. supper	ər	ɝ by most American speakers and ə by many others
16. bird	ûr	ɝ, ɜr by most American speakers and ɜ by many others
Phonemic Diphthongs		
1. I'm	ī	aɪ
2. how	ou	au or ɑu
3. annoy	oi	ɔɪ

individual sounds of the blends are under control. Typically, younger children omit one of the sounds or substitute another which is, for them, easier to produce. *Drink* may at first be produced as *dih* and later as *dink* or *dwink* before the child gives it a "grown-up" pronunciation. In the same way, *please* may begin as *pee* and then become *pease* before it becomes a word of four sounds and the *l* is included in its proper place.

Many children, in their early efforts at articulation, reverse the order of sounds. *Ask* may be pronounced as *aks*. A favorite pronunciation is *pasghetti* for *spaghetti*. Some of these "cute" sound order reversals become family words. But there is a danger involved: The child may be embarrassed when using these words outside the family, as he or she may be misunderstood, or laughed at even when understood.

COMMON ARTICULATION ERRORS

Most of the articulation errors that children have follow a certain pattern. Here are a few guides that may help parents decode their children's messages:

- Sounds such as *k* and *t* are often interchangeable; so are *d, b,* and *p;* and either *t* or *k* and *d* and *g*. In a child's early speech attempts, one of these sounds may be used for any of the others. Thus, *candy* may be *pandy* or *tandy*, *tick-tock* articulated as *dik-dok* or *dod-dod*
- A sound used in one part of a word may be used again in another part of the word. So, *dolly* may become *doddy*, *kitty* may become *titty* or *kicky*, and *Fido* may become *dodo* or *fofo*.
- In general, sounds mastered at an early age are substituted for sounds mastered later. Table 4.3 may serve as a guide on this matter.
- Children perceive certain common combinations of words in a different way than adults do. They perceive them as they are in fact pronounced! So *an apple* may be heard as a *napple*. An early pronunciation may be *nappuh* before it becomes *napple*. Subsequently, the *n* is dropped and the *apple* emerges as the fruit of the articulatory labor.

What should I advise parents to do about such "errors"? My answer is, "Nothing directly in the way of correction." If the child hears enough examples of the adult form of any given word, he or she will eventually use the adult form. Usually, before the child begins to use the adult form, the child will reject the infantile pronunciation (mispronunciation) and so show that he or she is about through with baby talk. Just as the child manages to learn not to say *napple* unless saying *an apple*, he or she will also get the right order of the syllables of *spaghetti* and later of *elephant* and even *hippopotamus*.

Children straighten out their listening, their ability to keep a sequence

Table 4.3. Order by Average Age of
Consonant Sound Control*

Average Age	Sounds
2	h, m, n, w, b, p, t, k, g, ng /ŋ/, d
3	f, y /j/, s, r, l
4	ch /tʃ/, sh /ʃ/, j /dʒ/, z, v
5	voiceless th /θ/, voiced the /ð/
6	zh /ʒ/

*Correct articulation at least 50% of the time for a given sound
in two or three positions.

Note. From "When are Speech Sounds Learned?" by E. K.
Sander, 1972, *Journal of Speech and Hearing Disorders, 37,* p.62.
Copyright 1972 by the American Speech-Language-Hearing
Association, Rockville, MD.

of sounds in correct order, before they are usually able to correct their own pronunciations. Thus, even after a child knows whether the adult has produced the sounds and the syllables in proper order, he or she may for a while continue to produce a word with the sounds in a transposed order. However, if we take the word *spaghetti* as an example, a child may say *pasghetti* but refuse the food, or at least the pronunciation for it, if mother also says *pasghetti* to him or her but not to adults. (I assume that the *pasghetti* pronunciation has not become regularly used by all members of a family.) If the child does hear the correct pronunciation, in time the correct one will be produced.

There are some words that defy many adults. The word *ask* is pronounced *aks* by numerous older speakers. We have also heard highly intelligent and well-educated speakers pronounce *larynx* as *lar niks* and *pharynx* as *phar niks*.

By 18 months of age, most children make two important and related discoveries. Though what they hear from grown-ups is physically a stream of syllables punctuated by occasional pauses, sputterings, and bursts of sounds, somehow they discern that (a) a stream of speech has identifiable words, and (b) the words are made up of identifiable sounds. Before they make these important discoveries, adult speech must sound like jargon to them. Jargon is what we often accuse them of perpetrating. Just what is jargon?

JARGON AND THE REASONS
FOR IT

Jargon is a stage that often, but not invariably, follows the two-word level of language acquisition. Once children make the discovery that they can identify more than one word in a stream of utterances, they often become jargon speakers—that is, they imitate what they think (perceive) they hear.

Most adult speakers, quite properly, tend to emphasize the first and last "main" words of a sentence. Usually, these are the words we would retain if we reduced a message to an economical telegram. In most sentences they would include the subject (a noun or pronoun) and the predicate (a verb), and/or the object of the verb. A child might recall the phrase, "Johnny, have one of these nice cookies." At the two-word stage he might reduce this to "Johnny cookie." But, though Johnny may not recall all the other words he heard, he does recall that there were other sounds. So, usually with appropriate intonation, Johnny-the-jargon-speaker may fill in the places between *Johnny* and *cookie* with a production of unintelligible sounds that to him represent the flow of adult speech.

Not all children indulge in jargon, at least not to adults. Some speak jargon to their pets. Others speak jargon to themselves before falling asleep. Probably all jargon speakers reveal to us how we sound to them.

Moreover, jargon for its own sake may be fun! We can get some idea of how we sound to young children if we recall how foreigners sound to us when they speak to one another. They all seem to speak with amazing speed. They articulate faster than we can comfortably hear. When we learn a new language, even a few words of a language new to us, the speakers seem to slow down. Actually, it is our hearing–listening mechanism that has adjusted. Even for grown-ups, speaking jargon may be fun, otherwise we would have no songs that go "koo-koo-ka-choo" or "hey nonny nonny." Many of us, or at least our friends and neighbors, do talk admitted nonsense to pets and to children.

Parents should be aware, however, that not all that sounds like jargon is intended as jargon by the child speaker. The adult must try to tune in and do some articulatory decoding. The guidelines suggested above should help. One way of testing whether the child is using jargon intentionally is to respond with some jargon of your own. If the child seems pleased, then assume it is intended as sound-play jargon. If, however, the child becomes disturbed, angered, or frustrated at your inability to understand the message, it is *not intended* to be sound-play jargon. Then, it is the responsibility of a motivated adult to try some decoding. If you don't succeed at first, try again. If you continue to fail, find a better decoder, if one is available. If not, show your regret, change the subject by using a short utterance of words and sounds the child can produce.

Some children reserve their use of jargon for occasions that parallel those in which adults might swear, use nonsense language, or speak intimate love talk. That is, like adults, children produce jargon speech to express feelings and emotions for which they have no words. As children grow older, they too will emulate adults in their use of emotionally laden language. Like them, they will learn to say things that are biologically improbable and genetically incompatible and inconceivable. But until the child learns this earthy, largely Anglo-Saxon derived vocabulary, he or she has to be content with jargon.

INTELLIGIBILITY AND THE PARENT'S ROLE

Normally, the intelligibility of a child's speech increases with age. At the one-word stage, usually between 12–18 months of age, about 25% of the words are readily intelligible. The percentage is higher for adults and often for older siblings who are good at guessing. With a limited child vocabulary, guessing is not too difficult. In the two-word stage, usually between 18–24 months, from 50–70% of children's utterances are intelligible. By 3 years of age, almost all utterances can be easily understood. However, understanding a child's speech may still call for decoding or making necessary sound substitutions by listeners. Those listeners who are intimately involved with a child may do their decoding without conscious awareness of the process.

Normally, when children are 4 years of age, there should be little need for sound-substitution decoding. This does not mean that the child is at the adult level of proficiency in articulation. It does mean that, because the child is speaking with conventional grammar (or at least the grammar of older persons in his surroundings) and uses appropriate intonation, *messages as a whole are intelligible*, even though some of the child's speech sounds are still not up to adult level of competence. This, of course, assumes that the adults do in fact have proficient articulation.

What advice can we give to parents and other caretakers to help children toward intelligible speech? The answers are simple. Most parents and mature caretakers do these things quite naturally.

- When speaking to a preschool age child, speak in simpler sentences and more slowly than you would to a grown-up child or another adult.
- If a child is not proficient in sound production, do not reject attempts at speaking. Try to understand.
- Do not imitate the infantilisms that constitute baby talk. Be an adult. That is what the child expects.

In keeping with the suggestions above, let us suppose that a 2-year-old child says "Dada pay wadio." The response of the *dada* should be "Daddy will play the radio" or even more simply, "Daddy plays radio." If he enjoys being called a *dada* then, simply, "Dada plays radio." Then he should be sure to suit the action to the words. When the radio is on, he might then state "Radio is on," or "Radio playing." It won't hurt to exaggerate the *r* sound, but it should not resemble the growl of an angry dog.

Except by example, parents should not correct their children's speech. Comparatively few children have "defective" articulation as they mature. With good models, nearly all children who are born with the usual sound-producing and hearing equipment learn to articulate proficiently. Almost all so-called errors correct themselves by age 7 or 8. If a particular child does not become intelligible by then, despite good models, professional help is indicated.

A final caution to parents: Some children have several kinds of difficulty in speaking. They may have trouble in organizing their language, in finding appropriate words, and in using conventional grammar, as well as in articulating. If your child is like this, *do not correct his articulation.* This kind of child, even more than others, would be held back by being corrected. Excessive self-consciousness about speaking may produce an insecure, hesitant, halting speaker. Articulation may improve a little, but possibly at the expense of overall fluency. At worst, the child may become a stutterer. I will consider this problem in Chapter 5.

In the next chapter, I discuss children who continue to have unintelligible speech and an overall pattern that is often confused with stuttering.

In Chapter 9, I discuss a small but seriously impaired group of children who, in addition to severe speech sound deficiencies, are also delayed in initial comprehension and production of speech. This group is also markedly slow in progressing from single-word to multiple-word constructions and in grammatical acquisition. There is strong evidence that many, if not most, of these children are "brain different."

SELECTED RECOMMENDED READINGS

The recent literature on articulation disorders has been burgeoning, so has the literature on normal articulation development. Among recent publications that consider both aspects of articulation as well as the relation of articulation to overall language acquisition are the following:

Eisenson, J. (1984). *Aphasia and related disorders in children.* New York: Harper and Row, Chapter 7.

Eisenson, J., & Ogilvie, M. (1983). *Communicative disorders in children.* New York: Macmillan, Chapters 10–11.

Ingram, D. (1977). *Phonological disability in children.* New York: Elsevier.

Shriberg, L. D. (1980). Developmental Phonological Disorders. In T. S. Hixon, L. D. Shriberg, & J. H. Saxman (Eds.), *Introduction to communication disorders.* Englewood Cliffs, NJ: Prentice-Hall.

Van Riper, C., & Emerick, L. (1984). *Speech correction,* 7th ed. Englewood Cliffs, NJ: Prentice-Hall, Chapter 6.

Chapter 5

Dysfluency Disorders:
Cluttering and Stuttering

CLUTTERING

The Sounds of Cluttering

The diagnostic term *cluttering* is more often used by European physicians, who practice *phoniatry*, than by American speech–language pathologists. In recent years I noted an increased use of the term *cluttering* by non-European speech experts and an awareness that clutterers, children as well as adults, present a combination of language organization problems, articulation difficulties, and dysfluency that suggest stuttering, at least on a superficial level. Before considering diagnostic differences and similarities between stuttering and cluttering, we may gain some insights from the following case study.

A mother brought her son to me with an insightful complaint. She said, "Johnny doesn't seem to be sure of what he wants to say, but he seems hell bent on saying it." Fascinated by this evaluation of her child's speech, I asked for a description of how the child actually sounded when he spoke. The mother not only described the boy's speech, but also brought a tape recording to support her description.

Johnny, at age 4, sounded as if he were talking with a hot potato in his mouth. His words were "too hot to handle." Some words, usually the short ones, were repeated, and longer words were presented in fragments, often with the order of sounds transposed. At best, articulation was approximate. The sounds and the words did not flow. Instead, they seemed to come in garbled bursts and sputters, and sometimes there were pauses at unexpected spots. Often sentences and even phrases were left dangling, as if they were beyond the control of the child.

As I listened, I realized that Johnny's speech suggested cluttering. It was *repetitious, fragmented,* and *too rapid for the boy's ability to articulate.* Another cause of the child's lack of intelligibility was his poorly organized phrase and sentence structure.

Cluttering and Normal Dysfluencies

In normal speech and language development, almost all children have periods of hesitant, repetitious speech when they begin to combine words into phrases and early multiple-word sentences. However, except for the jargon stage, and with allowances for articulatory proficiency, speech production is intelligible. In contrast, the clutterer's speech is indistinct, garbled, and characterized by overall unintelligibility. Whole phrases are repeated; others are interrupted and fragmented, then repeated once more. The speech productions of the clutterer give the listener the impression of a poorly organized, uncontrolled flood rather than an interruption of flow, which is more characteristic of stuttering. Moreover, the cluttering child, unlike the stutterer, appears to be unaware of this manner of speaking.

Cluttering and Stuttering

Stuttering or stammering* may be considered a disorder of speech production that is lacking in normal fluency and is characterized by repetition of sounds, syllables, and often of entire words or phrases; by blocking, usually of initial sounds, syllables, or words; by prolongation of sounds; and frequently by "fragmentation" of phrases. With the possible exception of their earliest stutterings, most children are aware of their difficulty in producing fluent speech. Stuttering will be considered in detail later in this chapter.

It is evident from the descriptions and definitions of cluttering and stuttering that both disorders share several features. Because of this, many speech–language pathologists and European phoniatrists consider the two disorders to be basically one, a disorder of speech fluency. For example, Perkins (1977) holds that cluttering and stuttering are "two overlapping general terms. . . . Behaviorally, cluttering is a useful term for identifying problems of rate and rhythm; to the extent that includes problems of fluency, it overlaps stuttering" (p. 325). However, Perkins also recognizes that, in addition to dysfluency, "clutterers tumble erratically through their speech, blurring intelligibility as they go" (p. 326). The effect, in my own terms, is *scribble speech*.

Perhaps a key difference between stutterers and clutterers is in their responses and apparent attitude to their speech. I know adolescents and adults with a lifelong history of cluttering, but they never developed the

---

*I consider *stammering* and *stuttering* to be synonymous terms. *Stammering* is likely to be used in countries other than the United States.

anxieties, fears, and apprehensions that most stutterers entertain. Clutterers, unlike most stutterers, appear to be willing if not ready to talk and to talk at length. However, cluttering may be a "cousin" to stuttering. Both stutterers and clutterers may come from the same family tree. If their problems in oral language production have a genetic basis, the paternal side is the likely contributor.

The Clutterer's Family

Much of how Johnny speaks—the Johnny described at the beginning of the chapter by his mother—also characterizes considerable adult conversational speech. We often hear, especially if we listen, agrammatical and ungrammatical productions from speakers who presumably could speak grammatically and fluently if they took the time to organize their productions. But this type of organization and production is not the norm for conversational interchange. Moreover, rarely do adults provide so few cues in their phrasing and incomplete sentences as to make their intended meanings too difficult to guess and so, to understand. Those who are both agrammatical and unintelligible are, like our Johnny, clutterers. The impression they provide is that they have only a vague idea of what they want to say, have not quite figured out how to say it, but have a compulsion to try saying it.

Johnny had a background typical of clutterers. He began to speak at 26 months. He walked at 18 months but often fell. He bumped and still bumps into whatever is available for bumping. Almost everything is in his way. He cannot yet ride a tricycle. He can throw a ball, but nowhere close to the target. He has not yet made up his mind as to which hand he will use for throwing, picking up a block, or holding a crayon. Essentially, he is still an awkward child, but he wants to do things. When he moves, he seems to move "all at once and all of a sudden" rather than with considered and controlled movements.

How do Johnnies get this way? In almost all instances, they resemble other members of the family, especially on daddy's side. The cluttering appears not only in speech, but later in reading and writing. Writing is often as illegible—scribbled—as speaking is unintelligible. Words are left out and spelling is poor. Both the adolescent and adult clutterer give the impression of being loosely and tentatively assembled persons, awkward and imprecise whenever physical skills are involved.

Table 5.1 sums up many of the essential similarities and differences between clutterers and stutterers. In this table, I have anticipated some of the discussion in the section on stuttering that will come later.

Table 5.1. Similarities and Differences Between Clutterers and Stutterers

	Clutterers	Stutterers
Family history	May be present, especially on the male side	May be present, much more often in males than females
Onset of speech	Often delayed	May occasionally be delayed, but not as often or as long as for clutterers
Likelihood of awareness	Usually unaware	Often aware to level of anxiety
Feeling about own speech	"Benignly" indifferent	Fearful, anxious
Likely result of		
(a) speaking after instruction to be careful	Improves	Increase of stuttering symptoms
(b) interruption and reminder to slow down	Improves	Worsens; anxious, tense, blocked speech
Speaking with awareness of importance of situation	Usually improves	Usually worsens
Speaking when relaxed, at ease	Worse	Improves
Reading new material aloud	Better at outset	Worse
Reading familiar material aloud	Worse	Improves

Advice to Parents on Helping the Clutterer

What can we do for Johnny to help him overcome his cluttering? More than most other children, he needs good models—adults who speak slowly, with clear articulation and good phrasing. He needs adults who can speak as if they were proficient actors: clearly, and more slowly than they usually do in adult-to-adult conversation. He needs adults who can speak, like actors, in lines that are completely formulated so that a sentence begun will be a sentence done. The sentences should be short and the phrasing apparent.

The child who clutters almost always speaks better when speaking slowly. So, whenever Johnny-inclined-to-be-a-clutterer does speak slowly, be sure to respond *promptly*! Indicate your approval. Engage him in conversation, speaking slowly yourself. If the family is getting ready for a picnic and Johnny asks, "Where we going?" an appropriate answer is, "We're going on a picnic, Johnny." After this sinks in, you might then ask, "What would you like to eat?" When this matter is settled, you might then get to "What shall we take to play with?" or "What shall we play?" Short interchanges are better than an answer such as "Johnny, you see we're going on a picnic. We'll have lots of things to eat: eggs and cheese and hot dogs and cookies and crackers. Then we'll play, etc., etc., etc."

My experience with children who are clutterers or who are likely to be clutterers indicates that they tend to improve when they slow down and "mind their speech." They improve when encouraged to speak in short, complete sentences for which they have adult models. They improve if they are given visible cues when their speech becomes rapid or explosive. We suggest that parents tell children inclined to be clutterers "I'll touch my ear when you speak faster than I can listen."

Reading aloud to the child is helpful. Reading might begin with looking at books with no more than two or three pictures on a page. (You want an *uncluttered* page.) Say something appropriate and relevant about each picture. "The birdie flies," "The boy jumps," "The baby cries," matching each statement to the picture.* Then ask the child to tell you about the picture. If the child's words are intelligible, show your approval. If not, don't reject what the child says. Instead, ask, "Did you say the birdie flies?" and encourage the child to say it clearly, with a visible reward to follow.

Help the child build up a useful treasury of words and phrases related to the reading of pictures. Later, read simple stories. Read them at a slow but undistorted rate. Give Johnny things and happenings to talk about and the words for the things and happenings.

If the child is of school age and is showing evidence of being a clutterer, professional assistance is indicated. This assistance should be directed toward helping the child organize his or her thinking in words before speaking aloud. The child needs help to make simple statements simply and ultimately to become a slow and considered speaker. When the child grows up and does indeed sound as if some thinking generally precedes speaking, he or she will earn an enviable reputation.

Here are two final questions for parents of a child who clutters.

- Is your household one that does not suggest the need to hurry?
- Will you listen to Johnny if he takes his time to figure out what he wants to say, and will you patiently listen to him while he says it?

Reading for Meaning (Eisenson, 1984b) is a reading program that provides for the "reading of pictures" before the reading of words. The program proceeds, through illustrations and associated written language, to establish grammatical constructions in a sequence that follows normal acquisitions. This approach helps the child *to organize language* as he or she learns to read.

If the answers are yes and the parents do provide Johnny with good models in their own slowly produced, well-organized speech, then they are doing what they should. But a yes also means that the atmosphere and tempo of the home do not include haste and stress. Parents are responsible for whether a child who is inclined by way of inheritance to become a clutterer actually becomes one. In some instances, changing the atmosphere of the home helps the adults take life easier in a variety of ways, including their speech.

A relaxed attitude on the part of parents and a relaxed home atmosphere do not imply carelessness or looseness in thinking. Quite the contrary. Dr. Weiss, in his clear and concisely written, now classic book, *Cluttering* (1964), emphasizes that the clutterer is an imprecise thinker who must be helped to think clearly. He writes, "The clutterer's haphazard and tentative thinking in preparation for speech reflects his general approach to all undertakings. This is the basic characteristic of cluttering and hence one of the prime targets of therapy" (p. 36).

I have one note to add. Therapy should be a family affair. The goals of treatment are not limited to the child. They hold for all members of the family who fit the description of the clutterer.

STUTTERING

In the section on cluttering, in which I anticipated some of this discussion, I offered a tentative definition of *stuttering,* a term used synonymously with *stammering. Stuttering* was described as a disorder in which speech production lacks normal fluency and is characterized by repetitions of sounds, syllables, and often of entire words and phrases; by blocking, usually on initial sounds or syllables; by prolongation of sounds; and frequently by "fragmentation" of phrases. Most frequently, but not invariably, the speaker entertains apprehension and anxiety about speaking and shows evidence of "struggle behavior."

Because of the component of repetition and the suggestions of dysfluency, it is not surprising that parents of young children, those between 2 and 3 or 4 years of age, want to know "Is my child really stuttering?" The question may also be asked about children up to age 6 and, less frequently, up to age 9. Dysfluent speech characterized by repetition is almost universal in young children but stuttering affects only about one child in a hundred.

In this section, I consider how stuttering begins and how it develops. I also consider a normal manner of speaking that superficially resembles and is confused with the dysfluencies of stuttering. Advice and guidelines are offered on what parents can do to prevent normal, dysfluent child speech from becoming stuttering and to prevent incipient or early stuttering from becoming a chronic problem.

Transient and Chronic Stuttering

Except for the most facile speakers, all of us can recall occasions when we spoke dysfluently, with more than the usual amount of word repetitions and interspersed "uh uh" and "you know" and "I mean." At the moment of such dysfluent speaking, we may even have thought of ourselves as speaking like a stutterer. These occasions are frequently, but not always, associated with the need to say something about which we are not secure or certain. Sometimes, we need to organize our thinking and, at the same time, put our thinking into words for a listener. If the listener is someone we consider important, then the hesitations and the repetitions and the filler "words" and interspersed phrases become more frequent.

However, though an adult may momentarily regard this speech as stuttering, *he or she does not become a stutterer.* A stutterer is a speaker who is chronically apprehensive about his or her ability to speak without frequent self-interruptions. These fears are accompanied by self-criticism and anxieties that tend to turn the fears into self-fulfilling prophecies. Young children are not born with apprehensions and self-defeating attitudes, but they are almost all capable of acquiring them.

One of the confounding problems of stuttering is that it doesn't happen all the time. As we have not noted, nonstutterers are more fluent with their speech at some times than at others. Factors such as fatigue, stress, pressure for quick responses, and the importance of the listeners are likely to make all practiced speakers more hesitant. By and large, the situations that make nonstutterers less fluent are the same ones that make a stutterer more likely to stutter. Any factors that lead to normal hesitations and repetitions are likely to produce considerably more hesitation behavior in young speakers. And they lead to much, much more hesitation in children who are incipient (beginning) stutterers.

It is sometimes difficult to distinguish between normal hesitations and repetitions—normal dysfluencies—and incipient stuttering. Fortunately, there are other factors that can help us identify the child who is, or might be, an incipient stutterer and to distinguish that child from the normally fluent one, who nevertheless indulges in some hesitations and repetitions. They will be considered in a later section. Notice, however, that I have used the term *incipient stutterer* because no child, regardless of manner of early speaking or of background factors, which I shall soon list, needs to become a full-fledged stutterer. Parents need to be advised that the factors associated with stuttering do not invariably lead to stuttering. A child may have factors in his or her background that match those of stutterers, and so may be predisposed to stutter and still not become a stutterer. If a child has sensitive treatment and care, stuttering can be avoided.

Some Facts About Stutterers and Stuttering

Research about children who stutter has been going on in the United States, Great Britain, and other countries in the Western world for more than half a century.* Despite differences in points of view as to causes and even the nature of stuttering, there are some observations about which there is strong consensus and which I consider as facts.

- More boys than girls stutter. The ratio is about 3 or 4 boys to each girl.
- Stuttering tends to run in families. Families that include a stuttering child are more likely to have relatives who stutter than are families without a stuttering child.
- Families with twins are more likely to include a stutterer than families in which all children are singletons. Identical twins have a higher incidence of stuttering than fraternal twins.
- Stutterers are likely to be somewhat slower (later) in beginning to speak than nonstuttering children.
- Stuttering is almost always a problem of early childhood, as it usually begins between 3–9 years of age. Only rarely does a child begin to stutter in postpubescent years unless he or she, for however brief a time between the ages of 3 and 9, had shown indications of incipient or outright stuttering. Onset after age 10 is notably rare. The exceptions are children who may have incurred brain damage after a history of normal speech.

The literature indicates that stuttering may begin as early as age 2. However, unless there is a family history of stuttering, there is little likelihood that the hesitations and repetitions common at this age are true precursors of stuttering.

The Onset of Stuttering and the Organization of Language. How do we apply the information just presented to answer the question, "Is my child real-

---

*The literature on stuttering has been burgeoning since the 1920s. The recent literature has considerably more scientific research support than during earlier decades. I make no attempt to provide a survey of the literature but instead cite the chief sources that support the facts about stuttering. These can be found in the selected reading list at the end of this chapter and include the following: Andrews et al., 1983; Eisenson, 1975; Eisenson and Ogilvie, 1983; Howie, 1976; Kidd, 1980; Van Riper and Emerick, 1984; and West, 1958.

ly stuttering?" Again, I emphasize that, even if all the factors listed above fit a particular child's profile and even if the child is a "self-interrupter" and possibly an incipient stutterer, he or she need not inevitably become a chronic stutterer. However, I think that there is strong evidence that among children who are excessively dysfluent, and especially those who are self-interrupters, is a small population who have difficulty in learning the rules (grammar) of how words are strung together in conventional constructions we call sentences. Children seldom if ever stutter or repeat or fragment words when they are at the single-word stage of speech development. Perhaps the acceptance of built-in syllable repetition for the important first words, as in *mama*, *dada*, and *wawa*, make such syllable duplication acceptable. Most children continue with such syllable duplication or near duplication in their first vocabulary so that we are likely to hear *wow-wow* or *wow-wowi* for dog and *be-be (bay-bay)* for baby. However, by age 2 these infantalisms are no longer acceptable, especially when the child begins to produce utterances of two or more words. At that time, repetitions assume a negative value. It is often at this stage of multiword production and conventional (grammatical) organization that we are likely to get the dysfluencies suggesting the onset of stuttering.

If we understand the relationship between early dysfluencies, normal and excessive, and early language acquisition we should be able to advise parents and other caretakers on how to reduce the likelihood that incipient stuttering will develop into a chronic problem.

Many speech authorities, myself included, regard excessive dysfluencies and incipient stuttering as evidence that the child is slower in acquiring and organizing language than most children of equal age and intelligence. Almost all children are born with the capacity to acquire one or more languages and the capacity and related abilities to understand and produce speech.

But some are more proficient and gifted in this potential than others. Some children are early and fluent speakers, who begin to talk at 8 or 9 months and speak in full grammatical sentences by 15–18 months. Most children show these accomplishments a few months later. They start to talk between 12–15 months and speak in grammatical sentences between 18–24 months.

Children who stutter are likely to belong to the slow-average or somewhat late-to-start-to-talk group. Perhaps, if parents and other significant relatives would not look at these children with anxious expectation, if they would accept, at least initially, a limited degree of competence in talking as they do in other skills, we might have even fewer stutterers than we presently do. We don't expect all children who run to do the 100-yard dash in less than 10 seconds, nor do we expect all children who draw to become professional artists. But, in our culture, we do expect, not necessarily on a conscious level, that all children will become skilled in speaking. Moreover, we expect the skill to be established and manifest by the time the child enters school.

A slow-to-start-to-speak child, who is hesitant and repetitive, may not be at all slow in nonspeaking skills. But he or she is, no matter how intelligent and otherwise skillful, a "special" child. The child may be special in that for many years, perhaps into adult life, he or she will not be as prompt and proficient at organizing language as most other children the same age. The child may become a capable and even brilliant writer, as some of my colleagues have done who happen to be stutterers and may even become an excellent actor or public speaker, *providing the speech or lines* are carefully memorized. But, writing is usually done at one's own rate, and acting and public speaking rarely include impromptu and unrehearsed repartee. It is in the give and take of conversation that stutterers of all ages have their greatest difficulty.

In a pilot study of seven stutterers and an equal number of normally fluent children, ages 5.0–8.8 years, Stemach and Eisenson (1977) found that when the groups were compared in spontaneous speech, the stutterers

1. Made a greater number of single words statements.
2. Used simpler grammatical constructions.
3. Made more grammatical errors.
4. Had a greater number of errors of articulation.

Case histories of the stutterers revealed that they were about 2 months later in speech onset than the normally fluent children.

The implications of these observations is that a productive therapeutic approach with young stutterers, or with those who might be at high risk for becoming stutterers in the light of family background, would help them in the organization of their early language. Luper and Ford (1980, p. 264) note that "It has been our clinical experience that therapy designed to increase basic language skills frequently leads to a reduction in disfluencies in young children who stutter." Stocker (1976), in her *Probe Technique*, elicits responses on "levels of demand," which are in effect linguistic levels that increasingly require the organization and production of "creative" language. Dysfluencies increase with level of demand. This information is used by the clinician as a basis for helping the child organize and produce language with a minimum of dysfluency.

Normal Hesitations versus Stuttering

Earlier in this chapter, I contrasted cluttering and stuttering. Now, my contrasts will emphasize the differences between normal hesitations and repetitions (normal dysfluencies) and stuttering. A child may be considered to be stuttering if he or she has difficulty in organizing a flow of speech and expresses this difficulty by

- Abrupt hesitations
- Frequent repetitions of a single word, a syllable, or a sound
- Maintaining a "sticky" position of the speech articulators (the tongue, lips, or palate), or
- Any combination of these behaviors in speaking.*

At the outset, a child may not be aware that he or she speaks in any unusual way. Actually, it is just as well that the child lacks this awareness. When, all too soon, the child becomes aware that he or she is a different kind of speaker—a "different" child—defensive techniques to avoid speaking may develop. Or, the child may postpone attempts at speaking even as he or she starts. The child may, in effect, begin an internal struggle that gives subsequent speech the flavor of starting and abrupt stopping, and starting and stopping again.

But not all hesitations and repetitions are stuttering. Not all those who hesitate and repeat their words are necessarily even incipient stutterers. More than 99% of all children, adolescents, and adults engage in some degree of hesitation and repetition as they speak their on-going thoughts to another person. Let us call these hesitations and repetitions *normal hesitation behavior*. It is the way almost all of us speak when we are figuring out what to say to share our present and on-going thinking with a respected listener.

There are a few among us who somehow are gifted with supernormal fluency, who have the gift of gab. But most adults, and almost all children, show hesitation (dysfluency) behavior in up to 10% of the sounds and words they produce. Late adolescents and adults may do somewhat better. Some adults repeat and hesitate considerably more than most children, but they still are not stutterers. Most normal hesitations and repetitions are of whole words or phrases, or they are fillers such as *uh, uh* or *well, well, I mean*, or *you know*.

How then do we distinguish the stuttering child from the one with normal hesitations and repetitions? One distinction is in the manner of rhythm and flow of speech. Easygoing, "bubbly," and bouncy repetitions—even brief hesitations—do not noticeably interfere with the rhythm and flow of speech. In fact, repetitions may help the child maintain speech flow while figuring out how to share on-going thinking. Repetitions of this sort

---

*A "sticky" position is one in which contact between the articulators is excessively tight or compressed. To the listener, it seems that the child must exert great effort to break the contact and continue with the utterance.

usually occur on a full syllable, or entire word if it is a short one, or even on an entire phrase. So "I, I, I . . . " or "I wanna, I wanna, I wanna . . . " are not at all unusual ways for a child to start a sentence. "S, s, s, see" or "br, br, br, brother" is more indicative of stuttering. In general we may say that syllable repetition or any *broken word* repetition is in the direction of stuttering, while whole-word or short-phrase repetition is well within normal speech. However, either kind of repetition is suggestive of stuttering if it is accompanied by "sticky" positions or obvious tension of the articulators.

Prolongations—stretching out a speech sound—may also be suggestive of stuttering, especially if the prolongation is excessive and frequent and suggests tension. Again, almost all of us stretch a stretchable sound such as *m, n, s,* or *sh* occasionally. But if often for example, while trying to make up our minds as to the day of the week, we produce something like, "I'll see you *sss* or *s, s, s* you Sunday," or "I'll, I'll *s, s, s* sssee you Ssssunday." This is not usual dysfluency and very much in the direction of stuttering. In general, the longer and more frequent the speech production includes prolongations and "involuntary" repetitions, the more the speech is in the direction of stuttering rather than normal hesitations. If the dysfluencies have the appearance and "flavor" of tense or forced articulation, the greater is the likelihood that we are dealing with incipient stuttering.

At this point it is important to emphasize that I have known children between ages 2 and 4, and even older, who spoke for brief periods in a manner suggestive of stuttering *but who spontaneously became normally fluent and did not continue in the ways of stutterers*. Others, under conditions of tension, reverted to excessive dysfluency *but did not become chronic stutterers*!

Incipient Stuttering: Attitude and Treatment

What advice can we give to parents about their 2- to 6-year-old child who may be an incipient (early stage) stutterer? Let us assume that either by the child's manner of speaking or fear of speaking, the parents, and perhaps you as a consultant, accept that the child may be in the first stage of stuttering. In addition, the child's "profile" and family history reinforce the possibility that the child is, indeed, prone to stuttering. What the parents report and what you observe make you reasonably certain that the child is not demonstrating normal speech dysfluencies. He or she is not only hesitant and a self-interrupter but also a word fragmenter rather than a bubbly whole-word or whole-phrase repeater. The child is more likely to produce a dysfluent flow such as "muh muh muh Monday, I,

I, I'm gu gu gu going to school' rather than "Monday, Monday I'm, I'm going, going to school." Occasionally, he or she seems to prolong and with considerable force emit a sound like "mmmmmmmm Monday." Moreover, this young child has a cousin, with whom his family has had no face-to-face contact and who, at age 10, is a stutterer. So stuttering may run in the family on a hereditary rather than contact basis.

The first bit of advice I give to parents is to get rid of the idea their child, even if excessively hesitant and repetitive, will inevitably become a stutterer. A predisposition to stuttering and even indications of incipient stuttering do not mean that the child is certain to become a full-fledged stutterer! If, however, the parents, or an older brother or sister, or some other key member of the family does anything to make the incipient stuttering child anxious about speaking, chronic stuttering may be the consequence. As a formula of probability, stuttering is most likely the result of excessively dysfluent behavior plus awareness plus anxiety plus not knowing what to do about producing more acceptable speech. In contrast, dysfluent speech without awareness or anxiety is likely to remain within the range of normal speech production. Accordingly, parents must do all they can to ensure that the child's speech, no matter how dysfluent, is accepted and acceptable while the child learns more about language, preferably with the help of good examples.

I advise parents not to look at their child with evident anxiety and so express fear that their child's words may not come out free of hesitations and repetitions. I remind parents that almost all adults occasionally show evidence of hesitation. If they are doubtful, I may record and play back a conversation with them. I also recommend that they tune in on a radio or TV honest-to-goodness spontaneous interview or a talk show and to note the amount of dysfluency produced by professional performers who presumably are normal or superior speakers. I also remind parents to make sure that everyone else who has contact with the child—aunt, uncle, grandparent, teacher, or respected friend or neighbor—also cooperates in easing the child's self-consciousness about speaking.

I remind parents that their Johnny or Joannie, who is comparatively a newcomer to speaking, has even more right to dysfluencies than older relatives and professional speakers. Johnny, or Joannie, for that matter, did not learn to walk without considerable stumbling and falling. But very few Johnnies or Joannies, including those who are a bit awkward, become chronic stumblers.

I try to help the parents to an attitude of benign tolerance—an attitude of accepting what the child *can do* as a speaker. Really, there is no choice. Not to accept the child's speech is unrealistic and may produce the very behavior—stuttering—that they surely want to prevent.

I give parents the following lists of directives, Do Nots and Do's, to guide them if I suspect that the young speaker may in fact be an incipient stutterer. I would give them these same lists if the parents believed their child was becoming a stutterer, even though I may consider the child to be normally dysfluent (actually, normally fluent).

Do Not's

- Do not use the word *stuttering* or *stammering* or any equivalent term to describe your child's speech. If the child does hear such a word, he or she will want to know what it means—and *somehow* will figure out, no matter what you say, that it is not good to be a stutterer.
- Do not tell your child to slow down, to stop and think before speaking, or to "start over again and do it right this time." Nor should you say or do *anything* that will make your child feel or suspect that there is anything wrong with how he or she talks.
- Do not look at your child anxiously, afraid that the word flow may not meet your hopes for fluency. Neither should you sigh in relief when the child does somehow manage to speak without the usual hesitations.
- Do not ask the child to speak if he or she prefers to engage in some other activity. If you make a mental note, or a written one, about situations that are associated with an increase in hesitation behavior, you can avoid asking or expecting your child to speak in such situations.
- Do not discourage the child from speaking on any occasion when the child wishes to talk. If you can, however, "control" the overall environment so that the child will not feel a need to talk in the situations where, as you have noted, he or she is likely to be excessively hesitant or repetitious.

Do's

- Establish as tranquil a home environment as you can achieve without suppressing other members of the family. Try to avoid or reduce the need for speaking in stituations that have heightened excitement or produce frustration (as in some games). Children need to learn to live with and accept occasional frustration. But they do not need to talk during or immediately after experiencing it.
- Listen to your child with full attention and patience. When Johnny is talking to you, attend to him at least as much as you would like him to attend to you when you are the speaker.
- Speak to your child in a calm, unhurried manner. However, do not slow down so much as to be "dragging out your words" or with an absence of normal rhythm. Occasionally, your speech should include an easy, bouncy repetition, if only to demonstrate that anyone, even a parent, sometimes indulges in hesitation behavior.
- Keep your child in the best possible physical condition. Illnesses are likely to bring on an increase in hesitation behavior. Expect this and accept it if it happens.

- Expect that your child, like many adults, may have a greater urge to speak than to say anything in particular. Joannie may start to say something when she has neither the thought, the words, nor the sophisticated devices to complete her utterance.

  If your child starts something he or she cannot finish, smile pleasantly and let the child off the hook. One way is to ask an easy question or make an observation to which the child can readily respond. The question or observation should have some relation to the situation the child is talking about, however, and this may require a bit of creative thinking. Your question or observation may refer to an earlier part of the conversation.

  Thus, if the conversation with Joannie or Johnny included talk about a game, or a child with whom she or he was playing, you might refer again to this event or child.
- If your child appears to be groping for a word, or for a turn of phrase to complete a statement, wait a decent time for the word or phrase to come. If it does not, calmly and casually provide the word of prhase. If at all possible, do so by using the word or phrase in a statement or question of your own.

  This technique has the added benefit of providing a complete-sentence grammatical model that your child may imitate. With practice, the child may even make it part of habitual speech behavior. But remember that children (and adults, too, for that matter) are likely to be most dysfluent when learning and trying out new words and new verbal constructions.
- Although you should casually provide a word or phrase when your child needs it, don't be in a hurry to jump in and obviously complete your child's thoughts. Give the child a chance.
- Do all you can to make speaking pleasurable. Engage in "party talk," but talk as an adult. Don't talk down to the child. Tell short, amusing anecdotes and play riddles, especially ones the child can guess correctly. Read to your child, especially at times when you have noted that your child is likely to speak with increased hesitation behavior. Your child will learn that there is pleasure in listening as well as talking.
- If your child asks whether there is anything wrong with the way he or she speaks, or demands to know, "Why can't I speak right?" assure the child that he or she is speaking "right." If the child insists that "sometimes my words don't want to come out," explain that you know and that this happens to you, too. It happens to everyone. Do not go into long explanations, however, that reveal your own anxiety. Most children can easily tell when their parents are worried about something.
- If you need help in understanding or following these directives, consult a competent speech or language clinician in your community. Be

sure that the person you consult is qualified and competent. If you are in doubt, write to your state hearing and speech association or to the American Speech-Language-Hearing Association (10801 Rockville Pike, Rockville, MD, 20852).

Stuttering Among Children in the Early School Years

The early school years, ages 5–9, are also the years in which stuttering is highly prevalent. Some of this is "confirmed" stuttering, among children who were more than normally dysfluent as early as age 2. Others were not so identified but showed evidence of "full-fledged" stuttering, beginning at ages 6 or 7. A smaller percentage showed their first strong indications of stuttering at ages 9 or 10. These children, regardless of identified age of onset, have in common a production of speech characterized by excessive repetitions, hesitations, sound and syllable prolongations, word fragmentations, and blocks. In many instances, they also engage in "struggle behavior," which appears to the onlooker to be an effort to break the block and so move on with the speech effort. Also common to this population is awareness and accompanying anticipation and anxiety about speaking.

Whether or not the children have insight about the nature of the speaking situation that is conducive to their stuttering, they do not alway stutter but they nevertheless are apprehensive that they might. As a general rule, the amount of stuttering varies directly with the meaningfulness—the informational content—of the message and especially so if the message (statement) has to be organized by the child. In effect, the child has the responsibility for what and how his or her words are to be chosen and delivered. It is likely that the early school years emphasize this responsibility. What can we do for these children?

Advice for Parents of Early School Age Stutterers. First, I emphasize that the treatment of the young (school age) stutterer requires professional attention and not the advice of neighbors, relatives, or friends, however well intentioned they may be. Second, the treatment of young confirmed stutterers should involve all of the grown-up members of the family as well as the child. Parent counseling is a must.

When I counsel parents of stutterers I have two objectives in mind: (a) to provide information about stuttering and children who stutter, and (b) to provide opportunities for relieving parents of their feelings of guilt, anxiety, and hostility, both self-directed and child-directed. Parents no less than children need and deserve time and opportunity to express their feelings, their fears, and their hopes. These burdens should be addressed and shared with an understanding professional person, who knows how to listen, remain objective, and respond according to need.

Here are some of the things I try to share with parents:

- Even a "confirmed" stutterer does not necessarily become a chronic stutterer.
- Stuttering is often an "on again" and, fortunately, "off again" phenomenon. If the parents can keep a diary of the situations that turn stuttering on, they may help to keep it off.
- Children who stutter are likely to increase their stuttering under any form of stress. This includes the stress brought about by awareness of a need to communicate, to deliver a particular message. Communication cannot, of course, be avoided, but the stuttering child should not be pressured or hurried to deliver the intended message.
- Conflict between the stuttering child and a parent, or older sister and brother, is conducive to stuttering. It is hardly surprising that such conflicts are often replay of differences and disagreements that the parents of the stutterer had with their own parents.
- Permissive attitudes are likely to reduce stuttering. Rigid, perfectionist ones are conducive to stuttering.
- Almost all children who stutter are able to speak easily and fluently when they pretend to be someone else, when they "act." This is especially so when the child can memorize words and play out a role.
- Children who stutter usually have no difficulty in speaking in chorus (two makes a sufficient chorus), or in singing, or in reciting from memory.
- Children who are confirmed in their stuttering should be encouraged to speak in situations in which they can be relatively fluent. In this way, they may learn that there are situations about which they don't need to be apprehensive. The best way for parents to impress their children about their fluency (no-stuttering) situations is to look approving—a smile will do—*after the child has been fluent.* Do not make a big thing about it. If you do, the wise child may conclude that he must be a mighty bad stutterer at most other times.

Although it is now too late to prevent the onset of stuttering, it is not too late to help the stuttering child. Those who can help are the parents, the clinicians, the teacher, and the child himself. With early intervention, the secondary characteristics, which are a consequence of the child's reactions to his or her stuttering, can be avoided or minimized. It is essential that the cooperative treatment efforts be in the hands of a professional person who specializes in the treatment of young stutterers. The American Speech-Language-Hearing Association can provide a list of such specialists, certified speech pathologists, throughout the United States. The

Canadian Speech and Hearing Association can do the same for clinicians in Canada.

SUMMARY AND PROSPECT

It is important to distinguish between normal dysfluencies and those associated and predictive of stuttering. If stuttering persists, then many of the problems that generate from stuttering will also require treatment. These include generalized anxiety and fears about speaking, struggle in the initiation of speech, and possibly phobias about places, persons, words, and sounds. We also find some stutterers who become experts in the use of techniques and tactics to avoid speaking but who are not so expert in avoiding feelings of guilt and a lack of self-worth. These are all secondary characteristics that develop as reactions to stuttering.

High priority should be given to preventive treatment for children who meet the "criteria" for those who are at high risk for becoming stutterers and show evidence of incipient stuttering or who are early-age stutterers. Such therapy should emphasize helping the child to organize language in keeping with our present knowledge of normal child language acquisition. The young school age child who is excessively dysfluent or who stutters may also profit from such instruction. The prevention and treatment of stuttering are family affairs. Parental counseling is an integral part of the treatment program.

Finally, some words of caution. The literature on stuttering and stammering is vast and, especially to the layperson, often quite confusing. In our present state of knowledge, no cure can or should be guaranteed. Books by self-acknowledged experts who promise cures should be avoided. On the other hand, books and programs by qualified authorities who consider how stuttering behaviors and attitudes can be modified and controlled are another matter.

I have selected several books and sources from which to obtain information about stuttering and stutterers that are written in language that can be understood by professionals who are not in the field of speech pathology as well as by laypersons. The selection does not pretend to be all inclusive.

SELECTED RECOMMENDED
READINGS AND RESOURCES

Andrews, G., et al. (1983), Stuttering: A review of research findings and theories circa 1982. *Journal of Speech and Hearing Disorders, 48,* 226–246.
Bloodstein, O. (1975). *A handbook on stuttering,* rev. ed. Chicago: National Easter Seal Society for Crippled Children and Adults.   This booklet

provides a review of research and theories on stuttering. It includes a chapter on treatment.

Bluemel, C. (1957). *The riddle of stuttering*. Danville, IL: Interstate Publishing Co. This book, written by a psychiatrist, is deservedly a classic. To solve "the riddle of stuttering," Dr. Bluemel distinguishes between stammering and stuttering. Stammering is poorly organized language that becomes disorganized, and so stuttering occurs under stress. Therapy emphasizes the need to help the child in the organization or reorganization of language. Bluemel held that "talking is thinking out loud." Accordingly, he directed attention to the thinking process in speech, which he considered to be of greater importance than the talking process. "The mind broadcasts to the mouth. The words say themselves."

Eisenson, J. (Ed.). (1975). *Stuttering: A second symposium*. New York: Harper and Row.

Eisenson, J., & Ogilvie, M. (1983). *Communicative disorders in children*. New York: Macmillan. This textbook includes a chapter on *Stuttering*. It emphasizes problems in stuttering in the school age child.

Howie, P. M. (1976). The identification of genetic components of speech disorders. *Australian Journal of Human Communication Disorders, 4*, 155–163.

Kidd, K. K. (1980). Genetic models of stuttering. *Journal of Fluency Disorders, 5*, 187–201.

Speech Foundation of America, Malcolm Fraser, Director. P.O. Box 11749, Memphis, TN. This organization publishes the results of meetings of authorities on stuttering in booklet form. The information provided is concise and written in layperson language.

Van Riper, C., & Emerick, L. (1984). *Speech correction*, 7th ed. Englewood Cliffs, NJ: Prentice-Hall. Chapter 8 reviews the development of the disorder in the child. The authors offer suggestions for treatment that includes parent counseling.

Van Riper, C. (1982). *The nature of stuttering*, 2nd ed. Englewood Cliffs, NJ: Prentice-Hall.

West, R. (1958). An agnostic's speculations about stuttering. In J. Eisenson (Ed.), *Stuttering: A symposium*. New York: Harper and Row.

Chapter 6
Vocal Disorders

In this chapter, I first explore some of the factors that influence a child's speaking voice; its melody and "musical" quality or its possible harshness, its nasal or possible metallic quality, the presence or absence of its lilt or its mellowness. Not all children are capable of qualifying for the poet's praise that, "Like music on the waters is thy sweet voice to me." However, with the exception of those who are born with atypical vocal mechanisms, everyone should be able to produce acceptable voice.

The characteristics that identify a child's voice begin to be evident when he or she is a tiny infant and posesses the innate capacity to distinguish human voices from other sounds. The child is born to be a listener before he or she becomes a speaker. Very early in life, an infant identifies and "echoes" the voices that he or she hears. But the echo is not really an imitation and remains the child's own voice. Despite changes with growing up, the voice will be readily distinguishable from that of other members of the family.

EARLY RESPONSES TO VOICE

Nothing is more distinctive in the behavior of infants than their responses to the human voice. Within the first few weeks of life, the baby will respond differently to the voice that purrs and the voice that snarls, to the happy voice and the angry voice. Very early in life, sometimes as early as 3 weeks, the baby may engage in a "dialogue of cooing" with a "cooing" mother. The baby may even learn to wait and take a turn. Angry voices literally "turn babies off." A baby may turn away from the voice or begin to cry. In contrast, the baby is "turned on" and toward the producer of the happy voice, especially if the happy voice is a familiar one. An unexpected voice may produce crying. The sound of the mother's voice may change the crying to cooing and later, when a child is more "sophisticated," to smiles and laughter.

The baby's early responses to the human voice are different from those to any other sounds or noises. We cannot be certain why this is so. It is

76

simply an aspect of what it is to be born a human being. Birds are responsive to other birds' noises, and so singing birds learn to sing. Dogs bark, cats meow, human beings vocalize and talk. Children who are born with normal equipment are "prewired" to be responsive to human voices. They are also equipped and constructed to make vocal sounds that are expressions of feelings: tender or furious, loving or hateful. They learn to use their voices to cajole or reject, seduce or repel. The voices of human beings can express subtleties beyond the meaning of words. They can even replace words when feelings or meanings cannot be verbalized.

The evolutionist Charles Darwin believed that this very human ability represents "an instinct of sympathy." Beginning in infancy and continuing throughout life, voice is the primary way in which human beings show their feelings and emotions. So the child, with an "instinct of sympathy," is in special tune with other human voices and uses his or her own voice to express feelings and emotions.

Bowlby (1958) considers crying and other forms of infant vocalization to be important attachment behaviors that are highly predictable in the desired outcome of bringing the mother or other caregiver to the child. Later, vocalizations serve to maintain interactions with significant others close to them. At a very early age, normal children learn that "dialogues" can be carried on through interchanges of vocalizations.

What do normal babies do with their voices when they hear the voices of significant others? Based on the investigations of Bruner (1975), Lewis (1951/1959), Wolff (1966), and others as well as my own experience, it is possible to make the following observations about the ways babies respond to voices:

- By the end of the first month, the baby cries when exposed to loud noises. The baby may make it a duet when he or she hears another baby crying.
- An adult voice, if it is not an angry voice, will have a soothing (quieting) effect on the baby.
- In the first or second month, the infant responds to a vocalizing adult by smiling. Often the baby will "hold a dialogue" with the adult, "cooing" back to the adult. The baby may start the "cooing" if the adult stops and so "keep the dialogue going."
- Children will "work" to hear a voice. One investigator, Dr. Sam Rabinovitch, measured the energy with which infants as young as 4 weeks suckled on a nipple while they were listening to recordings of their mothers' voices. When the voice recordings were stopped, the babies increased the energy of their suckling until the voices came on again. Then, the suckling energy went back to what was usual for the individual infant.

It is clear that the normal child needs to hear human voice and responds in different ways, according to what the voice expresses, very early in life. Favorable conditions, such as hearing human voices often, especially ones with soothing qualities, reinforce the infant's natural tendencies to vocalize. Conditions may also reinforce tendencies to be frightened or to be unhappy, if the baby's experiences are with unhappy or angry voices. These voices, of course, come from unhappy or angry persons.

The infant, or even the young child, cannot separate the voice from the vocalizer. The two go together in the child's mind, and either the person *or* the voice will make the child feel happy or afraid, as the case may be. Because children, especially bright children, tend to generalize their responses, they are likely to respond the same way to persons who are like those they already know, that is, respond in kind—with pleasure or displeasure, with joy or apprehension, with anticipation of security and comfort or with fear—to many persons who somehow individually remind them of the first person they associated with a certain feeling or emotion.

THE MELODY OF SPEECH

"All gone," says mother when the last spoonful of cereal has gone down the hatch. "Upsy baby," she says, when she picks up her baby. Each of these maternal exclamations is spoken with a melody appropriate to the words. So "all gone" is uttered as

all gone

and "upsy baby" as

upsy baby

Mother, by her words and appropriate speech "music," is teaching her child that there are patterns of melody or intonation that go with the flow of sounds.

Babies can usually distinguish between upward and downward melody (intonation) contours before they say their first words. So it is no surprise that their own first words are accompanied by melodies that they hear grown-ups speak. Some students of infant speech believe that babies are able to imitate adult speech melodies from 1 to 3 months before they say their first words, well before a year of age. These melodies extend a baby's repertoire beyond simple expressions of feeling and emotion. Preverbal vocal achievements are summarized in Table 6.1

Table 6.1. Early Vocal Responses and Productions Before First Words

Approximate Age	Baby Hears or Sees	Baby Responds
Birth–2 months	Loud noise	Cries
	Baby cries	Cries
	Eye contact with adult	Reflexively yawns, gurgles, coughs, sneezes; coos when content. May produce sounds such as *ayruh* when distressed.
	Angry voice	Baby cries and may turn away from voice.
	Nonangry voice	Coos in response
2–3 months	Sees face or hears familiar voice	Chuckling noise; laughter
	Unpleasant voice	Cries
4–5 months	Social play with adult. Tickling	Laughter, as for an older child. "Singing," cooing when child is alone and content.
6 months	Speaking person	Variety of vocal responses to indicate feelings. May "exclaim" to show delight. Child responds and imitates differences in vocal melody (intonation) patterns.
7–9 months	Presence of familiar person	Child's vocal contours (melody-intonation) suggest requests, demands. Sophisticated cooing expresses calmness and contentment.
10 months or earlier	Adult voice	Child responds by adjusting own pitch level in direction of the voice pitch of the adult, higher when responding to female than to male voice.
12 months	Significant other	Increasingly sophisticated vocalizations with communicative intent.

CAUSES OF VOCAL PROBLEMS

Identification and Imitation

Up to this point, I have considered the natural and intuitive way that babies and young children respond to the voices they hear. We have seen how they express their feelings, their frustrations, their contentment, and even their joy of being alive. In a very real way, babies reveal their budding individuality. We can identify the cranky, colicky baby through excessive crying. The calm, contented baby reveals personality through "dovelike" cooing. The lively baby earns a reputation through wide-ranged, happy-sounding vocalizing. The demanding baby has a voice that exclaims, commands, and demands loudly and assertively, with falling inflections.

I hesitate to say that "children are born that way," but they do seem to have natural tendencies. However, a voice pattern requires considerable practice and reinforcement before a mere tendency becomes habitual and a way of life. More often, it seems that children, because of an inborn capacity to identify and respond to human speakers and their voices, are "shaped" by the voices they hear. The chief "shapers" are their parents, older siblings, and other frequent caregivers. In most families the parents are the most significant caregivers. They are also, of course, the ones who may be concerned if their child's voice seems "to have something wrong."

In my own practice, assuming that I have medical clearance for the child, I ask the parents several direct questions. I emphasize at the outset that the questions are in the interest of the child. First, Have you ever heard your own voice as others hear you? The usual response is a surprised look. Then I explain that we hear ourselves through both bone and air conduction, while others hear us through air conduction alone. Unless we have had the benefit of a "candid" good quality recording of our casual speech and then an opportunity to listen objectively to the result, we continue to be strangers to the voice that others hear. I also urge that the parents make a separate recording of a conversation with an adult and one with the child about whom they are concerned. I ask that both recordings be brought in for comparison. The results are sometimes traumatic and most often revealing. We hear demands addressed to the child when requests would be more effective and certainly better for modeling. We hear sounds of irritation that are only in the recording of the speech to the child.

Then I am likely to continue, "Now that you have heard your own voice, what does it tell you? Do you like the overall effect? Is your voice unnecessarily loud? Is it hard, metallic, harsh, husky? Do you sound as if you're complaining, with whining tones? Or, does your voice sound as if you are making demands when you really intend to make a polite request? In speaking to the adult, did you sound apologetic or even self-demanding, when there was no cause or need for such an attitude?" In some instances I ask, "Is your voice thin rather than full? Do you sound as if you are almost out of breath?" Almost always I ask, "Is your voice in general—in quality, pitch, force, and intonation—the *you* that you truly want to express and convey? Most important, is your voice the kind that you would want the child you love to imitate?"

In my experience, both as a psychologist and as a speech pathologist, I have often had to make parents aware that it is not the child but the mother or father who needed treatment for a voice problem. On numerous occasions, I have pointed out to parents that their child must love them a great deal, because he or she sounded so much like them. And I proved the point with voice recordings. On most occasions, the way to treat the child was to treat the parents. Sometimes, just by listening to their recorded voices, parents were able to improve the quality of their voices in a direction more acceptable to them if they were listeners rather than speakers.

PHYSICAL CAUSES OF
VOICE PROBLEMS

Among the more frequent causes of vocal disorders in children are structural anomalies usually of the palate, disease associated with inflammation of the larynx and pharynx, the common cold, enlarged adenoids, and vocal abuse that results in changes of the vocal bands.

Denasal voice* is often a result of the nasal congestion associated with the common cold or allergies; enlarged adenoids produce the same effect. When a cold or other upper respiratory infection affects the back of the throat (pharynx) or the voice box (larynx) as well as the nasal passages, the result may be denasality and/or a harsh breathy voice. Any effort to produce a voice may often be accompanied by considerable pain.

Cleft Palate and Excessive Nasality

Palatal clefts and shortened palates are almost invariably associated with excessive (hyper-) nasality. Figures 6.1 and 6.2 illustrate such clefts. In general, any anomaly that permits "leakage" of air into the nasal cavities will produce a voice characterized by excessive nasality. A shortened soft palate (Figure 6.3) does not permit normal closure of the entrance to the nasal cavities and so also results in nasal voice quality.

Other Causes of Excessive Nasality

In some instances excessive nasal quality follows removal of the tonsils and adenoids because the child, to avoid pain, does not raise the back of the soft palate and the uvula and, therefore, does not "seal" the entrance to the nasal cavities. Any disease that weakens innervation of the palatal and/or pharyngeal muscles is also associated with hypernasality. Fortunately, now that poliomyelitis is under control this cause has become quite rare.

---

*For rather obscure reasons, many persons refer to the voice quality associated with a "stuffy nose" as *nasal*. This is both illogical and incorrect. When the nasal cavities, the chambers above the roof of the mouth, are clogged because of a cold or an allergy, the voice lacks nasal resonance and so is denasal. We can produce the effects of a denasal voice by pinching the nostrils and saying the sentence, "My mother may come to see me." The words may sound more like, "By bother bay cob to see be."

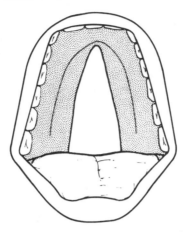

FIGURE 6.1. View of a child's mouth showing an incomplete cleft palate. The anterior portion of the hard palate and the gum (alveolar) ridge are not involved.

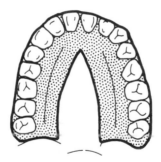

FIGURE 6.2. A partial incomplete cleft of all of the soft palate (velum) and most of the hard palate.

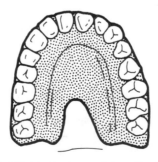

FIGURE 6.3. An incomplete soft palate.

If, after medical examination, neither a medical nor physical cause can be found for hypernasality, then the question needs to be asked, who is the child imitating? The answer might be a parent, a sibling, a playmate, or a respected older person who, despite his or her voice quality, is the child's role model.

Vocal Nodules

Thickened vocal bands and vocal nodules are among the frequent causes of hoarseness in children. The children so affected, more frequently boys than girls, are likely to be active, and sometimes hyperactive, energetic children, who are competitive in their play and do not spare their voices. High-pitched screaming gives way to breathy hoarseness because the child, to avoid pain, does not bring the vocal bands close together in speaking or in continued but failed efforts at shouting. The characteristic vocal qualities of a child with vocal nodules are low pitch, breathiness, hoarseness, and inadequate loudness.

Figure 6.4 illustrates the usual bilateral nodules formed on the upper third of the vocal bands.

Contact ulcers produce much the same vocal quality as vocal nodules. They are more likely to occur in adults than in children. Figure 6.5 illustrates the typical position of contact ulcers.

For detailed consideration of organic voice problems in children I recommend *Voice Problems in Children* (Wilson, 1979).

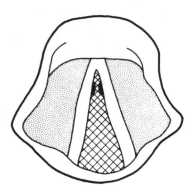

FIGURE 6.4. Vocal nodules, which are callous-like growths that typically form in the upper middle-third of the vocal bands. Vocal nodules are most often associated with high-pitched screaming.

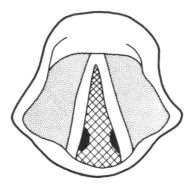

FIGURE 6.5. Contact ulcers. (Note the location at the lower portion of the vocal bands, in contrast with the position of the vocal nodules shown in Figure 6.4.)

Impaired Hearing

Functionally, *deafness* implies that, for a given individual, the capacity for hearing is so impaired as to preclude normal language acquisition. Nevertheless, deaf children, as well as adults, vocalize when they spontaneously express feelings and emotions. Those deaf children who are taught to speak tend to have voice characteristics that result from their failure to monitor the vocal components of their speech: excessive loudness, a higher than normal range of pitch when compared with their hearing peers, uncontrolled alterations in pitch, inappropriate nasal reinforcement (both hypernasality and denasality), and a voice quality that overuses back of the throat reinforcement (Boone, 1983; Ling, 1976; Wilson, 1979). The last characteristic, excessive pharyngeal resonance, is referred to as *cul-de-sac voice*, presumably because the back of the tongue is habitually raised (lumped) into the lower portion of the pharynx.

Children with lesser degrees of hearing impairment, the hard-of-hearing who can monitor their voice and speech, do not share the voice qualities of the deaf. Children with low-frequency hearing loss, who can benefit from amplification, can learn to monitor their vocal efforts and so have relatively normal voices. However, those who are hard-of-hearing and do not learn to monitor their vocal efforts demonstrate marked variations in nasal resonance, along the lines of the deaf.

Medical Problems

Children who lack physical vitality, and who are chronically tired are likely to have weak, flat voices (narrow in range of pitch and loudness). Children who suffer from endocrine imbalance may vocalize in too low or too high a pitch range, the direction depending on the specific nature of the problem. These vocal deviations are considered by Strome (1982) and Boone (1983).

In some instances, the voice of a child suggests and/or recalls a medical problem that no longer exists. A thin, flat voice that tires a listener may be a carryover of the child's habits that gained attention and advantages when he/she was ill. If, after medical evaluation, this is the case, then vocal therapy and possibly some kindly psychotherapy is in order.

At the risk of being repetitive, I again emphasize that no child should be given vocal therapy *without medical evaluation and clearance.* If at all possible, the evaluation should be made by a laryngologist.

ADOLESCENT VOICE CHANGES

Thus far, my emphasis has been on speech and language disorders of preschool and primary school age children. However, because frequently boys and sometimes girls have voice problems when they reach adolescence, I must consider this stage and aspect of voice development and the problems in voice production and control that may relate to them.

Beginning at about age 12 or 13, boys' voices change markedly in pitch and quality; these changes are less marked in girls. In boys, the vocal bands (folds, cords) grow about one-third longer from early adolescence to adulthood; the vocal bands also thicken. Because the range of pitch of the voice becomes lower as the length and thickness of the vocal bands increase, the overall result is that the adolescent boy's voice drops about one octave. In girls, because the vocal band length and thickness increase much less, the change in pitch range is not nearly as great or dramatic.* There is, nevertheless, a significant change in the quality of the adolescent girl's voice. Normally, the voice is richer and fuller than in childhood. The "ring" of childhood is replaced by the mellowness of maturity.

While girls' voices change in richness and mellowness, most boys almost literally obtain new voices. Once they played with voices in the range of the violin. During adolescence they must learn to manage instruments that have a cello to bass fiddle range.**

---

*Adult men's vocal bands range from .88–1.25 inch in length. Adult women's vocal bands range from .50–.88 inch. The larger the vocal bands, the lower is the pitch.

**The analogy to string instruments may be misleading. The voice mechanism is really more like a wind instrument. The vocal bands (folds, cords) or "voice lips" are similar to the reeds of wind instruments. The cavities of the windpipe (larynx), throat, mouth, and nasal cavities reinforce the tones of the vibrating reeds or vocal bands. Air (breath), under the control of the musician or speaker, sets the reeds or vocal bands into vibration and creates the identifying sounds of the instrument or voice.

For a while, boys' voices may seem to be out of control. They may become hoarse and husky or breathy. They may "break" in pitch and become falsetto. Suddenly and unexpectedly, even to the boy himself, the voices may go from a preadolescent high pitch to a treble to a husky bass. In a very real sense, it is as if a familiar musical instrument has become defective. It is as if someone had placed the reeds of a bass instrument, such as an English horn, into one intended for a considerably higher pitch range, such as an oboe, without informing the musician of the change. The instrument is literally out of tune. But worse, the reeds as well as the body of the instrument go on changing even while the instrumentalist is trying to adjust his techniques for playing it.

Most of the changes in voice are completed within a 6-month period. However, for a variety of reasons, including some that may be psychological, the changes or the adjustments to the changes may go on for a year or more.

Advice for Parents

What are the parents' responsibilities for the boy or girl whose voice is "not right" 6 months or longer into the period of obvious physiological adolescence? Usually, sympathetic understanding is enough on the positive side. Teasing, even when allegedly good humored and "for fun," is definitely to be avoided. If the adolescent's voice seems to be settling down, with fewer breaks and fewer uncontrollable changes in pitch and quality, then all the parent needs is patience. What should be happening is happening and all is going well.

Suppose, however, that either the boy or girl is trying to sound like a preadolescent child. The voice tends to be a falsetto, high in pitch, but without the quality of the child's voice. This may suggest that the physically adolescent boy or girl may still want or need to be a preadolescent child. I strongly recommend, however, that this possible conclusion *not* be made by the parents or any other relative. It should be made only by a *physician who understands young adolescents and their growing-up problems.* Parents should seek advice of such a physician. If the physician recommends counseling or psychotherapy, this advice should be followed. But the parents must assure the adolescent that he or she is not abnormal or neurotic or in any way sick, but rather needs help to get over this voice problem.

If the physician sees no indication of any growing-up problem, the adolescent may be helped by a voice therapist who *specializes in the speaking voice.* Let me emphasize the need to obtain medical clearance from the boy's or girl's physician, or from a laryngologist, before any voice training is undertaken.

In general, even when there are no serious problems, parents need to keep in mind the close relationship between voice and emotions in their adolescents.

Voices reflect slight changes in stress, and adolescence is a period of stress. The voice that reflects this state of feeling is not abnormal. If any treatment is indicated at all, it should be to help reduce stress. If reducing stress is not possible, an attitude of understanding will help. We do not need to verbalize this understanding unless the adolescent asks for it. A sensitive adolescent will be aware of the attitude and be grateful for it.

When the adolescent has learned to control his or her vocal muscles and has learned to adapt to the changes in the vocal mechanism, he or she will be able to control the vocal pitch and quality. This may take from 6 to 18 months. Patience is needed, both by the parent for the adolescent and by the adolescent for himself. Less frequently it may be for *herself*.

The vocal mechanism is essentially a wind instrument. As children, we learn to play the tiny instruments fairly effectively if we have proper models. As adolescents, we may have to learn again how to play the instruments. And again, as in early childhood, a poor model may make it difficult to adjust to the instrument or to attain an effective voice. But most of us, somehow, become fairly proficient vocal instrumentalists, at least for speaking, and all goes well. A fortunate few become virtuosos and learn to produce voices that are both effective and beautiful.

In the absence of physical or psychological problems, almost all children are capable of developing a moderately effective voice. Such a voice should be appropriate to the age, sex, and physical features of the child, the adolescent, and ultimately the adult. An acceptable voice should:

- Be pleasant, or at least not unpleasant, to hear.
- Reflect changes in feeling and thinking through pitch range, loudness, and quality.
- Be produced without discomfort and fatigue. However, fatigue and discomfort may set in with prolonged speaking.

I encourage parents to ask themselves, "Does my voice meet these criteria for acceptable vocalization?" If not, in the interest of their adolescent child, would they consider help to make it so?

The subject of adolescent (pubertal) voice changes is treated in Boone (1983), Greene (1980), and Wilson (1979).

Chapter 7
Brain Differences and Attention Deficits

STRUCTURE AND FUNCTION OF THE BRAIN

Although the structure of all normal brains is organized according to a general pattern, no two brains are organized precisely the same way. Differences may cause only slight variations from "normal" functioning, but in individual cases, minor structural differences may cause appreciable differences in functioning. Any of the factors such as dominant modality and manner of instruction, the age of the child when exposed to a given kind of instruction, maturation of given areas of brain, development of cerebral dominance—alone or in combination—may produce physiological differences in the organization of a brain that result in functional differences in behavior (Damasio, 1981). Thus, a child may develop patterns of cerebral connections that would be atypical for the population as a whole, or even of a subgroup of peers (left handers, for example) because of the particular way the child was taught or trained to perform a specific function at a critical age. By *critical* I mean at an age, usually before puberty, when the brain is highly impressionable, plastic, and not rigidly lateralized.

THE CHILD WITH MBD

The so-called minimally brain damaged (MBD) child, more likely the minimally brain different (MBD) child, is probably one whose brain has a difference in structural organization that causes more than a minimal difference in language learning. He or she is also one with attention deficits and, more often than not, is hyperactive.

Kinsbourne and Caplan (1979) use the term *cognitive style disorders* instead of *attention disorders* to refer to both overly impulsive and overly compulsive behavior. "*Extreme* impulsiveness is also sometimes called *hyperactivity* or *underfocused* attention. Extreme compulsiveness may also be called *overfocused attention*" (pp. 3–4).

In regard to possible etiology for these attention (cognitive style) differences, Kinsbourne and Caplan note:

> We know in principle that a lag in cognitive development can derive either from an individual variation in genetic programming or from early damage to an area of the brain destined subsequently to control the behavior in question. In an individual case, we sometimes have enough information to estimate the probability that one of these two general mechanisms is at work, but we have no available procedures that can incriminate either one with certainty. . . . From the therapeutic point of view the distinction is . . . academic, since knowledge of antecedents does not select more effectively from the range of therapeutic options. (pp. 8–9)

The description of a child that follows is illustrative of many of the behaviors associated with children who, by neurological evaluation, are confirmed to be brain damaged. In the instances to be presented, there was no neurological confirmation, but the behaviors were all there!

> Bobby is a wall climber! He is constantly on the go, disturbing everything he touches, and he touches everything within his reach. And little seems to be beyond his reach. For fleeting moments Bobby pays attention to everything within sight or hearing, but rarely does he pay enough attention to anything. Sometimes, however, he becomes compulsively involved with a toy or a block of wood or a piece of colored paper and concentrates on it beyond adult understanding. Bobby appears to have unlimited energy and wears out the adults who care for him. Bobby can't sit still or stand still until he is asleep. Yet, with all the energy he has expended during his long day, Bobby doesn't seem to need much sleep. His parents, unfortunately, do.
>
> What keeps Bobby and the adults who look after him on the run? And why is Bobby likely to be slow in beginning to talk, and later in learning to read and write and in learning what most children readily learn at school? With all the problems Bobby presents, to himself and to his family and teachers, the likelihood is that Bobby is not a mentally retarded child. He learns some skills remarkably fast, even if they are only the skills of knowing how to get what he wants, to move fast, to get into places he doesn't belong. Somehow we get an intuitive feeling that Bobby is a canny youngster who *learns on the fly and knows considerably more than he can tell, or cares to tell.*

Other Designations for the Child with MBD

Educators who may have been more concerned with the problems of learning rather than an often unsupported medical diagnostic designation substituted the term *dysfunction* for *damage*. A more recent term, especially for children who do not learn despite presumably adequate intelligence and normal sensory abilities, is *specific learning disability*.

The third edition of the *Diagnostic and Statistical Manual of Mental Disorders (DSM-III)* provides several related categories of developmental disorders that include or overlap the preceding designations (American Psychiatric Associations, 1980).* These encompass language, speech, and learning disabilities. In broad outline, they are

- Attention Deficits
  With hyperactivity
  Without hyperactivity
  Residual
- Developmental language disorder
  Expressive type
  Receptive type
- Developmental articulation disorder
- Developmental reading disorder
- Developmental arithmetic disorder
- Mixed specific developmental disorder
- Atypical specific developmental disorder

LANGUAGE AND THE BRAIN

I offer the following explanation to parents of children with MBD on how the brain functions relative to language and to learning that requires language. My emphasis is on how the brain, and particularly the cerebral cortex, functions in processing (comprehension and production) verbal behavior. Admittedly, it is an elementary explanation but not a misleading one.

Functional Differences Between Brain Hemispheres

The brain or cerebrum is divided into two halves (hemispheres) that superficially are more alike in appearance than most identical twins. But there are differences in structure that are related to differences in functions and responsibilities. The hemispheres are different but, in significant ways, still related, as shown if Figure 7.1. For example, both hemispheres have areas concerned with sound: the left hemisphere, for almost all of us, deals with the sounds of spoken language; the right hemisphere, with processing nonspeech sounds, such as mechanical noises, music, and even nonspeech human sounds. When we learn the words and music of a song, the left hemisphere learns the words and the right hemisphere learns the melody.

---

*My impression is that the *DSM-III* categories are over-inclusive. On a purely semantic basis, I have a problem with a category that is at once *mixed* and *specific*.

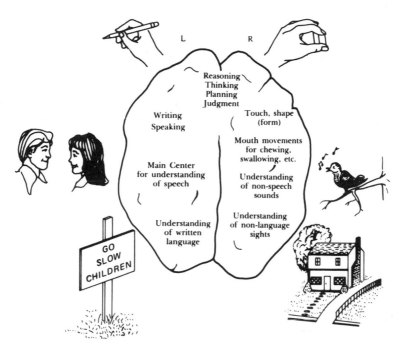

FIGURE 7.1. Differential functions of the cerebral hemispheres at the level of the cortex with special attention to the language areas (left half) and the non-language areas (right half). Although superficially the two hemispheres are almost identical in appearance, there are anatomical (structural) differences that are related to functions. We may note from the diagram that many of the functions are related as to intake modality. *Note.* From *Communicative Disorders in Children*, 5th ed. (p. 114) by J. Eisenson and M. Ogilvie, 1983, New York: Macmillan. Copyright 1983 by Macmillan. Used with permission.

Visual images are received by areas in the back of the brain cortex. The right hemisphere area is involved with images that do not require verbal decoding. But if the images are recognized as written words, their interpretation (reading) requires the specialized function of the left hemisphere.

As another example, the movements for chewing and swallowing are controlled by an area towards the front of the right side of the brain cortex. Movements for speaking, however, are controlled by an area similarly located on the left side of the brain.

Cerebral Dominance for Language

Note that, in all these examples, the left side of the brain is normally the one involved in language functions. This is so for understanding and producing speech, as well as for learning to read and write. Almost all right-handed adults have this kind of control or dominance for language.

Left-handed persons represent an interesting minority. About 50% of all left handers appear to have language functions, and probably other functions as well, controlled by either or both hemispheres. The other 50% seem to have control or dominance on the left side, about the same as right-handed persons.

The controls or dominance for language is established about the same age that children show clear preference for handedness. Thus, though one is not the cause of the other, hand preference and brain dominance for language develop together. By age 3 most children are clearly either left-handed or right-handed. A very small percentage are truly ambidextrous; that is, they can use either hand with almost an equal degree of skill. Another very small percentage are almost equally *unskilled* with both hands. In this small population, we find children who are slow in acquiring speech. We considered some of them in our discussion of cluttering.

Cortical Circuitry

The brain cortex contains billions of nerve cells, or neurons. Some of these cells are specialized and concentrated in areas or centers for special functions, as already noted and indicated in Figure 7.1. Other cells serve as conductors of impulses from one center to another and from one hemisphere to the other. Thus, we can talk about what we see, imitate the sounds we hear, monitor the sounds we produce, or even reproduce the sounds of the images that are stored in our minds.

The brain cortex makes sense out of sights and sounds. It is like a huge computer and switchboard that can deal with what our senses take in. It also enables us to organize the movements needed to produce our own sights and sounds, whether walking, running, speaking, writing, or whatever else a human being is capable of understanding and doing.

THE CEREBRAL CORTEX: ATTENTION, JUDGMENT, REASONING, AND PLANNING

The cortex of the brain is, at least up to now, the crowning achievement in human development. If the crown has any one area that makes it possible for us to behave humanely as well as humanly, it is the area in the front of the brain. The front or forebrain is larger in the human being than in any other primate. This area is responsible for planning, for exercising judgment, for reasoning, and for appreciating the consequences of our behavior.

In the forebrain, we make decisions, such as ''If I do this, the consequence may be. . . . '' In the forebrain, we do our planning, including most likely the planning of a sentence to be spoken or written. There also, as we have indicated, we can anticipate what may happen if we say something or write something. The forebrain is the ''If I'' or ''Suppose I'' portion of the brain.

What happens if this area is damaged by injury or disease? The results, known from actual cases, is a disturbance in the planning, judgment, and reasoning abilities.

Suppose, and now we speculate, that the frontal brain area does not develop on schedule. Then we may have an impulsive child who acts without regard to consequences. We may also have a child who is slow in acquiring speech because, as I have indicated, every word to be spoken requires the execution of a plan. For speaking, or for writing, the plans determine what sounds or letters constitute words, and what words are to be selected in a particular order to make a sentence. All this is in keeping with a master plan called *language*. Children with damaged or underdeveloped forebrains have a difficult time during any of this important planning.

THE CHILD WITH MBD
WHO DOES NOT TALK OR
IS SLOW TO TALK

About 30% of all hyperactive children can be diagnosed as having actual brain damage. These children are at the extreme. But moderately hyperactive children are not brain damaged, at least by medical standards. As we suggested earlier, they are probably brain different. What kinds of behavior do these children demonstrate? Most of them show the following:

- They usually are well within the average or above-average range of intelligence. This finding is supported by several psychological studies.
- They have trouble paying attention, especially to the words that people say to them.
- They are often impulsive and frequently difficult to control.
- They may be awkward and slow in developing body skills, including walking, running, hopping, and climbing.
- They are likely to be slow in developing skills such as building with blocks, managing a crayon, or dressing themselves.
- They are very slow in understanding language and in learning to talk. Some who do learn to talk may have difficulty in learning to read and write.

These children with MBD who have difficulty acquiring language represent a very small percentage, really a fraction of a percent, of all children. Some will pay attention quite appropriately to the sounds of pets and to mechanical sounds but seem to ignore speech. This may be explained by our knowledge that nonspeech sounds, including those made by so-called talking birds, are "processed" in the right hemisphere of the brain. Speech, as we have learned, is usually controlled or processed in the left hemisphere. Such a child may be telling us, by the sounds he pays attention to and by those he seems to ignore, that his left hemisphere had not matured sufficiently to be able to decode human spoken language.

In an extreme case, a child like this may be designated as *aphasic*, or nonspeaking. If the problem of language learning is not severe but retarded, the child is said to be *dysphasic*.* Fortunately, we know considerably more about such children than we did when their mothers were children. Fortunately, also, a considerable amount can be done for them by direct teaching of small and selected units of language. These units have been used in programs that parallel the speech development of normal infants and children. One such program is explained and illustrated in *Aphasia and Related Disorders in Children* (Eisenson, 1984a). I will consider aphasic and dysphasic children in Chapters 8 and 9.

However, I urge parents not to come to hasty conclusions about whether their child is aphasic or dysphasic. These children and their parents are entitled to professional evaluation and assistance from medical, educational, and language personnel who specialize in child language problems.

Why Some Children with MBD
do not Talk or are Slow to Talk

Now let us consider why children who are brain damaged (this condition determined by a competent physician) behave the way they are likely to. I say *likely* because one of the outstanding characteristics of these children is their quick and often frequent changeability. Further, we know that some brain-damaged children seldom if ever behave the way that most other brain-damaged children frequently do.

Damage to the cortex of the brain often produces extremes in excitability. At one extreme, the child is in a constant state of excitement, responding or attempting to respond to everything within sight, hearing, smell, or touch. At the other extreme, the child may respond to almost nothing; the child stares off into space or is excessively sleepy.

---

*The term *dysphasia* is generally used in Great Britain and Europe for hearing children, presumably within the normal range of intelligence, who are nevertheless significantly impaired in the comprehension and production of language.

Another effect of damage to the brain cortex may be a compulsion to continue responding to just one thing, one event, to the exclusion of all others. The child's attention may become limited to something the adult considers trivial: a piece of string, a block of wood, or a button on a shirt or dress. Nothing that is important (at least from the adult's point of view) enters the child's awareness.

For a child to acquire language, to learn to speak, the child must be able to pay attention to a speaker long enough to decode what the senses have taken in. If the child's attention span is too brief, if he or she pays attention for just a moment to everything but not long enough to any one thing, the child cannot take much into the mind nor store it there. If little or nothing is stored in a mind, there is little or nothing to remember and recall. So, in an extreme case, the child will not be able to learn the language and will not speak.

However, I caution parents that some children who are constantly on the go pay attention to considerably more than we give them credit for. They seem, literally, to learn on the fly. They do learn language, but seem to be too busy to speak to anyone.

Within the entire population of brain different children (not just those that are brain *damaged*) are a fair number who are slow in developing hand preference. They also seem to have trouble dealing with experiences that require them to take things in through more than one sensory avenue at a time. Sights that make sounds, such as a bell, may be disturbing bcause the child cannot readily make the correction between sight *and* sound.

We can only speculate that the reason for this is that the nerve cells or fibers that connect the brain centers for sight and sound may not be adequately developed. The timetable for the normal functioning of the specialized brain centers, and that of the conduction fibers, may be delayed compared with that of most children of the same age and potential intelligence. If there is an asynchrony, brain different children take in experiences differently, respond to them differently, and learn differently.

ADVICE FOR PARENTS OF
AN MBD CHILD

What parents should do for a hyperactive, distractible, MBD child is a matter that requires highly expert and specialized advice. By all means, parents should consult a physician and, if possible, a pediatric neurologist. In many instances, hyperactive children benefit from medications *that are prescribed and carefully supervised by a physician*. Highly specialized education should also be considered, and parents usually benefit from counseling as soon as the child's basic problem is identified.

If the child with MBD does not understand speech by 18 months at the latest, or understands spoken language but is not speaking by 3 years of age, preschool education with emphasis on language learning is in order. Many schools now have such programs.*

This discussion of hyperactivity and its *possible* implications may be anxiety producing for some parents, including those who may have come for a consultation about a child who has already been labeled *hyperactive*. Before the label gains the prestige of a diagnosis, several questions need to be asked: When is the child hyperactive? What is your basis for comparison, for deciding that the child is hyperactive? Hyperactive compared with whom? Under what circumstances? Many children, boys more often than girls, become fidgety (hyperactive?) when they are expected to attend to a situation beyond their period of interest and span of attention. They may, in fact, have obtained all that they want out of the situation. Their fidgeting and restlessness indicate that they are ready for something else. But their parents and later their teachers, may be working on a different time schedule.**

In consultation with parents I remind them that almost every child is hyperactive (restless) on some occasion. Waiting to go somewhere or to start playing a promised game are typical situations that generate restlessness. Unless the occasions are so frequent as to be beyond generous limits of expectation, there should be no cause for anxious concern. However, occasional and unexpected expressions of excitability should be noted. If such episodes increase in frequency, medical consultation is in order. Chronic hyperactivity may be an indicator of MBD but it need not be. Especially if the child is not or has not become deficient in learning.

Parents also become anxiously concerned about a child who, perhaps because the world is too much with him, ceases to pay attention to an expected situation and becomes compulsively involved with something trivial. This may be an indication that the child needs to "turn off" from environmental demands and "recuperate" from excessive intake. It may be a needed "time out" period. If, however, such behavior becomes frequent and chronic, then medical consultation is in order.

To sum up, children appropriately diagnosed as MBD require highly specialized professional attention. Experience indicates that most children with MBD benefit from specialized educational programs and some from

---

*Public Law 94–142, The Education for All Handicapped Children Law, mandates that school systems are to provide educational opportunities in the least restrictive environment for every child, regardless of handicap. Children with learning disabilities are included under this law.
**Ross. (1980, Chapter 13) reviews the literature on studies of presumably hyperactive children. In one study 49.7% of boys in kindergarten and primary school classes were described by their teachers as "restless and unable to sit still." This percentage would suggest that restlessness is the norm.

medical treatment that reduces hyperactivity and enhances attention span and opportunity for learning. Such medical treatment should be supervised by the prescribing physician. I remind parents that there are many causes and many possible treatments for children who are brain different. The diagnosis, and certainly the treatment, should not be made by the parents or by any relative or friends, unless they are professionally trained. Even then, it would be wise to make a referral rather than to make the diagnosis.

Information Intended to Be Reassuring

No matter what term is used, brain-different children are not necessarily brain-damaged, though about 30% of them may be. But many brain-different children are "off-schedule" in the development of expected behaviors, of which language acquisition is at the outset most prominent. Unfortunately for brain-different children, adult expectations are governed by what most children do, and not by what brain-different children demonstrate that they can or cannot do. Fortunately, most brain-different children, including those designated MBD, catch up. Their cerebral centers develop functional circuitry and their capacity to deal with events that come to them through all of their senses also catch up. For some children, catching-up may occur by 8 or 9 years of age, and for many more, just before they reach their teens.

SELECTED RECOMMENDED READINGS

Positions on minimal brain damage and its possible implications for "minimal" brain dysfunction have undergone considerable change in the period between the 1960s and the 1980s. The references that follow reflect some of these changes.

Clements, S. (1966). *Minimal Brain Dysfunction in Children*, NINCDS Monograph No. 3. Washington, DC: U. S. Department of Health, Education, and Welfare.   This monograph reviews the research on children with presumed minimal brain damage. Though a technical publication, it is not too difficult for the layperson to understand.

Ludlow, C. L., & Doran-Quine, M. E., (Eds.). (1979). *The Neurological Bases of Language Disorders in Children: Methods and Directions for Research.* NINCDS Monograph No. 22. Washington, DC: U. S. Department of Health, Education, and Welfare.   This technical, multiple-authored volume reviews recent research and projects research needs on brain and language functioning, normal and disordered, in children.

Psychology Today (November 1985).   This issue contains several articles written by authorities in their fields, on the brain, its structures and functions, with particular attention to language. The questions of left-handedness and differential brain functioning and sex differences in structure and functioning are also considered.

Ross, A. O. (1980). *Psychological Disorders in Children.* New York: McGraw-Hill.   Ross is a behavioral psychologist who has considerable reservation about the underlying implications of the terms *minimal brain damage* and *minimal brain dysfunction.* Attention deficits and hyperactivity are viewed as behavioral manifestations and educational matters, not necessarily problems. "Any intervention aimed at reducing hyperactivity must include a systematic plan to replace the hyperactive behavior with goal-directed, attentive, and constructive behavior."

Sanders. D. A. (1977). *Auditory Perception of Speech.* Englewood Cliffs, NJ: Prentice-Hall.   Chapter 9 deals with attention strategies, normal and faulty, related to language acquisition in children.

Wender, P. H. (1971). *Minimal Brain Dysfunction in Children.*   The author, a pediatric neurologist, presents an "older" view of the child with MBD. He emphasizes that "among children with normal intelligence and with good school experience, MBD is a very frequent source of academic difficulty."

Chapter 8
Delayed Language Including Hearing Loss and Autism

In this chapter, I will review and integrate information presented earlier with the specific objective of answering the question, "When is language acquisition significantly delayed?"

ORAL LANGUAGE ONSET

Speech is word-of-mouth language. Words consist of the sounds and combinations of sounds used in a particular language system, such as English, French, or Chinese. The forms of the words, the selection of sounds that produce meaning, are different for each language. The rules that determine how words are arranged in a sentence are known as *syntax*. A child who is delayed in speech may either not understand the language code or may not speak, even though it is clear by the child's behavior that he or she understands the language.

Obviously, we do not expect newborn infants to understand us. We do not consider them delayed in speech despite their profound inability to understand us or to make themselves understood beyond their urgent biological needs. But the time does come when we expect babies to understand some of the things we say to them. The time also comes when we expect them to use their mouths for something besides eating, crying, gurgling, and laughing. When should this time be?

If infants were statistics, I could answer this question with considerable assurance. In Chapter 2, I noted that some children (more likely girls than boys) say their first words before the end of the first year. A small percentage may even use words to name a few objects or persons as early as 8 or 9 months. But most children do not say intelligible words until they are 12–15 months of age. A few do not begin to talk until they are almost 24 months old. And a very small percentage may not say their first words until they are 30 months of age.

Who, if any of the children in these age groups, shall we consider delayed? Certainly not the children who understand speech and say their first words by 15 months. Is 2 years of age considered delayed? Perhaps, because purely on the basis of statistics most children, meaning more than 50%, say their first words by 18 months. But a human infant should not be treated as a statistic unless we play the numbers game intelligently. There are late talkers just as there are late walkers, late jumpers, late tricycle riders, and late block builders. Fortunately, in adjusting to the numbers game we can take comfort from the fact that many "latenesses" run in families.

A child may start to speak later than most children of the same age and sex; nevertheless, if that child comes from a family in which daddy, granddaddy, and Uncle Joe had nothing to say (or at any rate said nothing) until 24 months or even as late as 30 months, there is no great cause for concern. If, however, the child does not understand sentences, especially simple sentences made up of words that name things and actions that are part of everyday life, I would be concerned regardless of the family. Even a slow starter should understand relevant-to-the-situation statements, such as "Open your mouth" or "Here's your dolly," and respond appropriately. A child may close his or her jaws more tightly than usual or poke at the dolly's eyes just to show how he or she feels, even though an adult may not consider this an appropriate response. But even negative behavior may reveal that the child really understands what was said.

The 18–24-Month Period

For most children, the 18–24-month period is critically important. Normally, during these 6 months, language development progresses at a pace not matched during any other comparable time period. A child may enter this stage with his or her first intelligible words and a total production vocabulary of 5–10 words. Toward the end of this period, the child may be producing anywhere from 50 to several hundred words. Moreover, the child who has a vocabulary of 50 or more words is usually able to combine slected ones into phrase-sentences. These may begin with "mommy up" or "baby eat" or "doggy bow-wow."

As the child's vocabulary grows, the phrase-sentences usually increase in the number of words. Productions such as *"girl fall down," "look in it,"* and *"me jump up"* may be heard. At the outset of this critical age period, the child refers to herself or himself either by the name used by others or as *me*. At the end of the period, the child understands *I* and the difference between *you, me,* and *I*. Children also show understanding that *I, me,* and *my* is a self-reference made by the speaker and *you,* and *your* refers to the listener. Autistic children have great difficulty in establishing these linguistic, pronominal usages. Most normal children learn these usages at about 2 years of age.

With these references to vocabulary size and word-phrase length (mean length of utterance or *MLU*), we have another way of considering and measuring language delay. I noted that most children with a basic vocabulary of about 50 words begin to combine words into phrase-sentences. Children who do not produce at least two-word combinations when their base vocabulary has reached 100 words should be considered delayed in language development.

Now we are no longer referring to age but to size and growth of vocabulary. This way of viewing language development and language delay takes care of the late-starting child. The physically and mentally normal late-starting child catches up with the earlier starters. The gaps close between 36 and 42 months. However, the very early starters, especially if they are children of superior intellect, are likely to stay out in front. The greatest difference will be the size of vocabulary and in their capacity to comprehend and deal with abstract concepts.

The 24–36-Month Period

For most children who speak their first words no later than 12–15 months of age and show the expected rapid progress in the 18–24-month period, the next 12 months are likely to reveal significant acceleration and maturation in their comprehension and production of language. During this period it becomes evident that the child has figured out the linguistic code, or codes if the home is bilingual. The child's speech indicates that he or she knows that people speak in utterances that have "rules." The child's utterances incorporate the rules (syntax or grammar) of the older persons to whom she or he is regularly exposed. Statements are likely to be as grammatical or ungrammatical as those of older siblings and adults. Moreover, although the child may not be as proficient in articulation as she or he will by age 6 or 7, almost all utterances are intelligible not only to those who know the child well, but also to strangers.

We now have another way to assess when speech is delayed. It concerns *intelligibility*, which I first considered in Chapters 4 and 5. It is important that we differentiate *distinct* from *intelligible*. A child may produce a target sound without proper articulation, omit a sound, slur an entire syllable of a word, or transpose syllables (*elephant* produced as *ephelant*), yet the sentence as a whole may be *intelligible*. If it is not, and we assume that the older person is not too demanding and unrealistic in expectations, intelligibility as such can be a measure of speech development.

Of course, good articulation and intelligibility are related. Speech that has sloppy articulation is both indistinct *and* unintelligible. But a child of

3 may be highly intelligible, even if he or she doesn't have all the sounds and sound blends of the language under control. When a child has a vocabulary of 1000 words or more (which may be around 3 years of age), we expect intellgibility, even though the child has not yet achieved complete control over all the individual sounds and sound blends.

Articulation: Speech Sound Production. When Johnny says "Two cookie," is it because he cannot produce a final *s* sound, does not hear it, or does not understand how plural words are formed? The answer may well be *yes* to all three parts of the question.*

Table 4.3 lists the average age and order of consonant sound control. The indicated ages for "normal" proficiency in articulation cover years 2–6, but some children may not be proficient for all sounds until 7 years of age. By proficient, I mean about as accurate as adults speak in social conversations. Although consonant sounds are controlled at different ages, all vowels are usually mastered by 4 years of age. Exceptions may be found in children who have a low frequency hearing loss.

Table 8.1 on articulatory proficiency shows the order and age of control beginning at age 3 and going up to 7 years of age. In studying this table, and Table 4.3, we must use a reasonable amount of latitude and flexibility before deciding whether Johnny or Joannie is really delayed in articulation. Early talkers are likely to be closer to the averages shown than late talkers. Boys are likely to articulate later than girls. Children who have the sounds *p* and *l* under control may have difficulty in combining those sounds to say *please*; they pronounce the word as *pease*. Similarly, *flower* may become simplified to *fower*. By age 8, most children have sound blends, including the triple blend *str* as in *street*, under control. Again, the late starter should be given additional time before we decide that he or she is really delayed in speech sound production. It is also important to appreciate that it is usually wiser to compare a particular child with other members of the family rather than with children of other families. Slowness in the control of articulation sometimes runs in families. A year behind age expectations is well within range of tolerance.

As a general rule, there is little cause for concern unless a child's errors of articulation have some physical cause or are part of an overall delayed

---

*There is a fourth possibility. If the dialect the child hears does not require the use of *s* as a plural in phrases such as *two cookie* or *three book*, then the *s* will be omitted. Similarly, the child may hear *he go* to indicate present tense and therefore not use the final *z* sound in this phrase as in Standard English. Children who are exposed to and use American Black English should be judged on the basis of their dialect. To a speaker of Standard American English, a child who speaks Black English may not "sound right," but the child may nevertheless be not at all delayed.

Table 8.1. The Consonants of American English:
Average Age for Control

Sound	Average Age	Sound	Average Age
m	3	r	4
n	3	s	4.5
ng	3	sh	4.5
p	3	ch	4.5
f	3	t	6
h	3	th (*thin*)	6
w	3	v	6
y	3.5	l	6
k	4	th (*the*)	7
b	4	z	7
d	4	zh (*measure*)	7
g	4	j	7

Adapted from *Certain Language Skills in Children* by M. C. Templin, Minneapolis: University of Minnesota Press, 1957, p. 53.

language problem. Most "garden variety" speech defects improve by age 7 or 8 without any help from parents or other concerned adults. However, evaluation of the situation by a competent speech clinician is always in order, if only to relieve the parents' anxiety.

ARTICULATION AND SYNTAX OF INFANTILE SPEECH

Some children persist in baby talk later than norms of expectation and beyond liberal range of tolerance. Even at age 7 or 8, they pronounce their words in ways we identify as infantile. Moreover, some children construct their sentences like those of much younger ones, using syntax considerably below normal anticipations. The two tendencies—delayed articulation and delayed syntax—often go together. The overall flavor of their speech productions is *infantile*. For example, we may hear a 4- or 5-year-old child say, "Me want that" or "Me want ball" instead of the more mature constructions. Figure 8.1 shows the usual relationship between articulation and the development of syntax.

However, it would be misleading to generalize that children who are delayed in controlling the sounds of their language are also invariably delayed in their use of grammar. This is definitely not so for most children who have difficulty with a single sound, such as s, r, or l, or even with two or three sounds that are normally not under control by age 6 or 7. Some sound blends, such as sk and sks, are often not controlled by adults

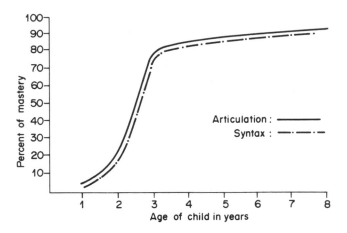

FIGURE 8.1. Articulation and the development of syntax.

who substitute a *t* for the *k* and say *ast* for *ask*. It does hold, however, that children who are seriously delayed in grammatical usage are also likely to be delayed in articulation. Some of their errors may, in fact, be grammatical rather than articulatory. The child who does not use a final *t* or *d* sound to indicate past tense, as in *we jumped* or *it spilled*, is delayed in grammatical usage rather than in speech sound control.

The child who says "He dwink wawa," when most children of the same age are able and likely to say "He is drinking water," is delayed both in articulation and grammatical usage. My observation is that the greater the delay in grammatical usage the greater the likelihood that the child will make speech sound errors even in single words. If a child's articulation and grammar both seem to be way behind those of other children of that age, then the parents should get professional advice. Investigators of child language are now of the opinion that significant deviations and retardations in phonology (articulatory development) may not just represent a speech sound disorder, but may be one aspect of a global linguistic disorder (Ingram, 1977; Menyuk & Looney, 1972).

CAUSES OF LANGUAGE AND SPEECH DELAY

Mental Retardation

The chief correlate and cause of delayed onset and development of spoken language is mental retardation. Nevertheless, all but the most severely retarded children acquire some speech. In general, the degree of slowness is related to the degree of retardation.

Impairments in development range from mild defects and slow onset in the mild or marginally retarded, to extreme deficits—total absence of communication through language—in the profoundly retarded. In their survey of the literature Carrow-Woolfolk and Lynch (1982) observe that "summaries of various surveys suggest that 100% of the profoundly retarded have impaired language, while 90% of the severely retarded (IQ between 21 and 50) and about 45% of the mildly retarded are so impaired" (p. 352).

In the most severely retarded, deficiencies in spoken language are often associated with organic anomalies and hearing loss. Lillywhite and Bradley (1969) surveyed several studies and found that educably retarded school age children have two to three times more hearing loss than do those of the nonretarded population. The percentage and severity of hearing loss increases in the more severely retarded.

It is interesting to note that those mentally retarded children, who do have language, develop their language system in a manner that is similar to that of normal children, *but at a slower rate* (Miller & Yoder, 1974).

Interestingly, by age 8 or 9, children who are mildly retarded are less different in regard to errors in grammatical usage than they are in the size of their vocabulary or in speech sound production. The grammar (syntax) that mild and sometimes even moderately mentally retarded children use is simpler in construction than the sentences of children with normal intelligence. An 8 or 9-year-old who is mentally retarded may say, "John is my big brother. He will take me to the zoo. We go tomorrow." These three statements are likely to be combined into a single complex sentence by an 8 or 9-year-old child of normal intelligence to "John, my big brother, will take me to the zoo tomorrow."

Hearing Loss, Impairment, or Hearing Handicap

Hearing loss (impairment) refers to the degree of insensitivity of the auditory mechanism (the physical deficit) associated with the loss of hearing. *Hearing handicap* refers to the response of the individual to the loss. Hearing handicap, though usually highly correlated with degree of loss or impairment, varies to some degree from individual to individual. It is possible for a child to have an objectively determined mild hearing loss and a much greater degree of hearing handicap. Conversely, in rare and fortunate instances, a child may have an objectively determined large amount of hearing loss, but in language learning and other behaviors, relatively small handicap is manifested.

Congential hearing loss implies that the impairment is a result of hereditary factors or consequences associated with birth. *Adventitious hearing loss* is an impairment that was acquired due to some disease or accident. The implications for such loss are quite different for a child who became deaf after learning spoken language, and who was once a proficient listener and speaker, from one who became deaf before learning to speak or shortly after the onset of speech. Some children, despite moderate to severe amounts of loss, show little evidence of difficulty in continued language learning or in school achievement following illness and hearing loss. Those who had not established speech as a habitual mode of behavior and a tool for learning usually need special education to learn speech and for academic achievement.

The hard-of-hearing are those who, despite degree of impairment, have functional hearing with or without the use of a hearing aid. Hard-of-hearing children learn to understand spoken language and to speak essentially in the manner of normal children; deaf children require specialized instruction in order to learn to understand and produce spoken language. Table 8.2 presents commonly agreed upon classifications and descriptive terms for amounts of hearing loss as expressed in decibels.

Central auditory processing disorders refer to the impairments in the perception and decoding of speech signals after they are transmitted to the brain cortex. This impairment will be considered in the next chapter, on developmental (congenital) aphasia.

Causes of Hearing Loss. Among the most frequent causes of hearing loss in children are heredity, infectious diseases such as meningitis and scarlet fever, and numerous bacterial and viral infections. Until fairly recently, maternal rubella (German measles) was a major cause. (The last major epidemic of rubella occurred during 1963–1965). Rh incompatibility is now a decreasing cause of hearing impairment.

Otitis media, probably the most frequently diagnosed illness in children

Table 8.2. Classifications of
Hearing Loss

Hearing Loss in Decibels	Usual Degree of Handicap
20–30	Slight
30–45	Mild
45–60	Moderate
60–75	Severe
75–90	Profound
90–110	Extreme

Note: From *Audiology*, 5th ed. (p. 360) by H. Newby, & G. Popelka, 1985, Englewood Cliffs, NJ: Prentice-Hall. Copyright 1985 by Prentice-Hall. Used with permission.

from birth to 3 years of age, may result in either transient or chronic hearing loss. Recurrent episodes of otitis media may produce permanent hearing impairment. Because this disease occurs so early in childhood, the consequences may delay the onset of language or cause long-term speech and language disorders. The sequelae of otitis media are considered in articles by Berko-Gleason (1983), Downs (1983), and Garrard and Clark (1985).

For reviews of varying effects of hearing loss in children, see Davis and Silverman (1978); Ginsberg and White (1978, pp. 8–22); Martin (1986); and Northern (1984). The publication *Childhood Hearing Impairment* (Canadian Minister of National Health and Welfare, 1984) includes chapters on prevention, evaluation, health services, and educational services available in Canada for children with impaired hearing.

Implications of Hearing Loss for Speech and Language. In general, hearing impairments have some implications for speech and language acquisition and deficiencies. Individually, as I have already noted, there are exceptions to the generalizations.

Unless the hearing loss is so severe that the child cannot learn speech at all by listening to others and to himself, the onset and development of speech are likely to be within the normal range. In general, children who are hard-of-hearing are likely to have more difficulty with articulation than with vocabulary and syntax. Difficulties in syntax are likely to be superficial. The child who cannot hear a final *s* or *t* or *d* sound may not be able to show a grasp of the notions of singular and plural or of present and past tense. A child may understand the statement "Three books are on the table," yet say "Three book are on the table" because this is what is heard. This example assumes that the omission of the *s* as a plural form is not due to dialect differences.

Children whose hearing is so severely impaired that they are considered deaf do not acquire word-of-mouth speech unless they are specifically taught. Some deaf children, even bright ones, have great difficulty learning to speak except through a system that includes visual signs (gestures, pantomime, and finger spelling). A combined system—a total method—that uses both signs and word-of-mouth speaking seems to be possible for many deaf children.

Assessment and Education of the Hearing Impaired. The medical diagnosis and treatment of the child with impaired hearing are the responsibility of an otologist. Assessment of hearing is the responsibility of the audiologist, a nonmedical professional. The audiologist also teaches the child to maximize whatever amount of hearing the child has, helps to determine the best type of hearing aid for the child who can use one, and teaches the child how to use and care for his or her hearing aid.

Education for the Deaf. How deaf children should be taught their language system and educated are lively issues in the field of deaf education. Methods of teaching language include the American Sign Language, newer sign systems that teach syntactical features of English, an aural–oral method that discourages signing and emphasizes facial (lip) reading and the maximum use of hearing with appropriate amplification, and a so-called total method that used both oral language and signing. Consideration of some of the involved issues are provided in Davis and Hardick (1981); Ling (1976); and Northern (1984). In any event, when the method by which a deaf child is to be educated has been decided, the overall instruction of the child is the responsibility of the teacher of the deaf.

Silverman, Lane, and Calvert (1978), who review the educational problems of preschool and elementary deaf, school-age children, are emphatic in their view as to the need for early education. These authorities are aware that deaf children, as a total special population, lag considerably behind their hearing peers at all levels of schooling. Specifically, "with the need to master new vocabulary and language, it takes about two or more years to achieve second-grade level and an additional one and a half years to complete the third grade." This delay "is not the fault of the child or teacher. It can be attributed to the time necessary to build a foundation for future progress."

PRIMARY AUTISM

A very small percentage of children seem unable to relate to and communicate with other human beings in normal and expected ways. The most extreme of these nonrelating children are identified as *autistic*. The failure of many of these children to learn to speak, or to speak in ways that are so idiosyncratic as to make for extreme difficulty in communication, almost defies comprehension.

The cause or causes of childhood (*early infantile*) autism are presently not known. The psychogenic position attributed to Kanner (1943), which viewed autism as an unhappy consequence of bad parenting and emotional neglect, is no longer taken seriously. Autism is now considered a developmental disorder that may result from neurochemical (neurophysiological) factors that involve the cerebral mechanism (Piggot, 1979). Essentially, autism is viewed as an organically based dysfunction of language and cognition that may be associated with perceptual malfunctioning (Schuler, 1984).

During early infancy, most children who turn out to be autistic do very little crying and are often considered to be "good babies." As they grow older, some autistic children show a special ability for humming melodies or reproducing songs, or repeating (echoing) strings of words that they hear but do not understand.

Autism is now considered a developmental disorder that is diagnosed and defined in behavioral terms (Ross, 1980). The absence or severe limitation of social and language skills for communicative purposes is the most prominent feature (Rutter, 1978). Some autistic children are "electively" mute for varying periods of time. A frequent idiosyncrasy of many verbal autistic children is the failure to learn to reverse personal nouns and pronouns, so that they refer to themselves by the noun or pronoun used to address them. For example, if the child is asked "Bobby, do you want a cookie?" the answer may be "Bobby want a cookie." If the child is addressed by, "Do you want a cookie?" the answer may be "You want a cookie." An echolalic response would be a repetition of the entire sentence (question) addressed to the child. However, a production that changes the intonation pattern from that used for an interrogative, *yes* or *no* construction to an appropriate declarative sentence intonation pattern would be an example of modified echolalia and have more favorable prognostic implications for future language development. Other features include abnormal responses to sensory input, ritualistic behaviors, and abnormal ways of relating to persons, objects, or on-going events in their environment.

Many, perhaps most, autistic children seem to have great difficulty in understanding that "speaking"—whether orally, by signing, by simple gesturing, or even by nonarticulate vocalizations that incorporate intonation patterns—communicates to others. In fact, even among autistic children who do speak, a striking, maintained feature is a *lack of evident communicative intent*. Some autistic children show limited communicative intent but fail to understand expressions of intention in those who address them. Schuler (1984) summarizes her position on the communicative ability of autistic children by observing that "communication problems reflect not only pragmatic but also cognitive failures, leading to problems of a magnitude that separate autism from other developmental language problems" (p. 261).

Mental retardation, present in varying degrees in many autistic children, further limits and complicates the communicative and cognitive aspects of childhood autism. Hearing impairment and central auditory dysfunctions, above and beyond peripheral hearing loss, are serious complicating factors for the development of spoken language.

Because many autistic children are characteristically echolalic, it is important to distinguish between types of echolalia. Whether echolalia is immediate, delayed, or mitigated (modified) has different implications for the development of cognition and communicative behavior (Fay & Schuler,

1980; Prizant, 1983; Schuler, 1984). In the next chapter, I compare child-hood autism with developmental aphasia.

Relationships and Models

Other relationship problems, less extreme than childhood autism, may be associated with language delay and improficient, slow language development. Any family situation that makes it difficult for a child to have a normal relationship with his or her parent may be associated with language delay and/or peculiar use of language after the child begins to talk. Children need to hear spoken language addressed directly to them as well as to overhear speech addressed to others. Normal stimulation should include simple, short sentences and simplified grammar *but not baby talk*. To be fair, parents and grandparents are entitled to some baby talk, but if this manner of talking persists, it is likely to maintain such speech in the child.

There is danger in too much talking as well as too little. A child overwhelmed with too much talking, some of which competes with radio or television or both, has a hard time making sense out of the "babble." Though most children from babble environments do somehow learn to talk, they do so despite rather than because of the help they get from older speakers. A little bit of quiet and some special adult-to-child speaking go a long way to help the child make sense out of speech sounds and, ultimately, to have a chance to say something independently.

Bilingualism

Are children who are brought up in homes in which two languages are spoken likely to be delayed in speech? The answer, if we are dealing with pure statistics, is yes. Yet we know that many children, perhaps even most children who hear two languages from the time they are infants have no difficulty understanding language or speaking. They are able to switch from one language system to another and may not even be aware that they are switching. But what of the statistics?

Studies indicate that an impressive number of children who are delayed in speech come from homes where two languages are spoken. Unfortunately, it is not always clear whether the adults have equal proficiency in both languages or are considerably better in one than the other. I suspect that equal proficiency is not the rule for the families of children who are delayed in speaking. Studies also indicate that children who are born into affluent bilingual families rarely have difficulty with understanding or speaking the languages they hear.

An old European tradition among the well-to-do was to hire a nurse who spoke a language other than the native one. The nurse spoke only her native language to the child she was helping to rear. Thus an advantaged child had two language experiences from early infancy. These children with bilingual exposure usually learned both languages without difficulty. We might conclude from this almost by-gone tradition that children from affluent homes, especially if the parents are high in intelligence as well as economic position, can learn two languages from infancy.

A somewhat safer conclusion is that a child should not be exposed to a second language until after he or she has achieved good control of a first. This age would be between 3 and 4. However, a child who has difficulty with a first language should, if at all possible, not be exposed to a second. Bilingual exposure for children who are slow starters and slow developers may cause confusion and more delay.

The recent burgeoning literature on the possible effects of bilingual environments on language development in children is not conclusive. Socioeconomic parental status, the proficiency of those speaking the languages, the status of the culture and the associated language are all factors that may influence a child's responses to the languages to which he or she may be exposed. I review the subject of bilingualism in Chapters 7 and 9 of Eisenson and Ogilvie (1984a) *Communicative Disorders in Children.*

SUMMARY

A child may be delayed in the onset of speech, in the development of vocabulary, in grammatical usage (the grammar or syntax used by older members in the child's special community) or in speech sound proficiency. "Average" children are what statistics are based on; in reality, children may deviate from statistics and yet fall well within the normal range when compared with other members of their families. "Normal" is a range, not a specific point. Family norms and ranges are often more relevant and individually more significant than large population norms. Therefore, the following observations are generalizations.

Children who are significantly delayed in language development are usually slow in all aspects of speaking. They are likely to be very slow in saying their first words, slow in learning how to put words together to form sentences, and slow in controlling the sounds of speech.

Children who are a bit on the slow side but have no physical problems or hearing problems and are of normal intelligence usually catch up in their delays by the time they are of school age; a few may need an added year or two to catch up. By age 8 or 9, most have caught up with other children of their age who were not slow starters.

Severely mentally retarded children may not progress beyond the use of single words. Their vocabularies may be limited to naming their basic needs. They say little because they have little to say. Yet it is significant that all but the most severely mentally retarded do speak in keeping with their needs.

Moderately mentally retarded children may not begin to speak until age 3 or 4. But if these children have no physical defects and have adequate hearing, their achievements in speech shadow those of normal children. They are slow in building up their vocabularies, in putting words together, and in speech sound control. But, after age 8 or 9, the most conspicuous difference is in the size of their vocabularies. Their sentences may also be more simply constructed than those of children of normal intelligence. A retarded child requires a separate sentence for each idea. A normal or bright child can incorporate several ideas into a single complex sentence.

Children who are unable to relate to speaking adults are very slow in acquiring speech. Some never do. Others speak, but in ways to express their feelings or nonfeelings rather than to share ideas.

Children with hearing loss do learn to speak. Some who are so severely hard-of-hearing as to be considered deaf cannot learn word-of-mouth speech unless they are taught by special methods. A few can learn only a visual language (sign, gesture, and finger spelling).

Finally, most children who do not acquire speech by exposure to normal grown-ups can be helped considerably by direct teaching. All but the most severely mentally retarded and emotionally disturbed can and do gain considerably from direct help provided by professional personnel. Where to find professional personnel will be considered in a later chapter.

Chapter 9

Identification and Differential Diagnosis of Aphasia and Dysphasia

IDENTIFICATION OF DEVELOPMENTAL OR CONGENITAL APHASIA

Developmental (congenital) aphasic children are the most severely linguistically delayed children who are not also mentally retarded or emotionally handicapped. In addition to their language impairment, these children also suffer from misidentification—by too many names and labels assigned to their "condition," and consequently, they also suffer misdiagnosis and inappropriate treatment. In addition to the term *developmental or congenital aphasia,** these children may also be labeled as *dysphasic* or *aphasoid*—terms that I recommend be reserved for children with less severe impairments than those designated as aphasic. Some professional colleagues, who prefer to reserve the term *aphasia* for acquired linguistic impairments, use the general term *severely orally linguistically handicapped*. Among the less fortunate misdiagnostic labels are *mentally retarded, autistic, childhood schizophrenic,* and despite evidence of ability to hear, *deaf*.

I recommend using the term *developmental (congenital) aphasic* for the child who, despite the conditions about to be listed, is severely delayed in both the comprehension and production of oral language:

1. Based on observation and if possible nonverbal assessment, the child appears to have adequate intelligence for the acquisition of spoken language.
2. The child has no abnormalities in the structure of the oral mechanism.

---

*I shall use the terms *developmental* and *congenital aphasia* synonymously to refer to those brain different children who are the subject of most of this chapter.

113

3. The child shows no evidence of early emotional or relating problems.
4. The child has no hearing problems except for spoken language. In this regard, the real problem involves listening rather than hearing.
5. The child's parents, or other caregivers, are available, willing, and presumably capable of providing normal opportunities and stimulation for learning spoken language.

ACQUIRED APHASIA AND RESIDUAL DYSPHASIA

The term *childhood acquired aphasic* should be restricted to those children who had acquired language normally and then, subsequent to identified cerebral pathology suffered through accident or disease, became impaired in language functioning. If the child improves and has only residual language and associated cognitive deficits, the diagnostic term should be *acquired dysphasic*, as is usually the situation when the cerebral pathology is limited to one hemisphere. These children will be considered later in this chapter. Thus, to establish a diagnosis of developmental dysphasia, the conditions just listed would be expanded to take into account the following considerations.

Adequate intelligence does not imply normal intelligence or normal cognitive functioning. Mildly, and even moderately, mentally retarded children learn to understand and, in turn, to speak the language of their environment. As a total population, most retarded children are more delayed in acquiring language than the nonretarded. Their speech is more often characterized by defects of articulation, voice, and dysfluencies than normal children (12% compared with 4.5%). However, their predominant deficiencies are in sparseness of vocabulary and difficulty in comprehending abstract meanings. But, as Benton (1978) observes, "there is also evidence that many retardates show pronounced impairment in the development of linguistic function that cannot be accounted for by their low mental age." Such children may be considered to be dysphasic-retarded.

Children with *structural anomalies* of the oral mechanism are not immune from the possibility of brain damage or brain difference that may also make them aphasic. However, the anomalies per se, such as cleft lip and cleft palate or deviant dental structures, would be much more likely to interfere with intelligible speech production than with spoken language comprehension.

There is no evidence that aphasic children have early emotional or relational problems; they relate normally to their mothers and other family members until they begin to acquire language. Therefore, emotional problems are more likely to be a reaction to failure in comprehension and language production than a consequence of initial abnormal relating conditions.

Hearing and listening must be distinguished for several reasons. Some aphasic children do have hearing losses of 15–25 decibels in the speech range. Such losses, ordinarily considered to be "mild," seldom cause language acquisition problems in the vast majority of children. Among aphasic children, however, this range of loss compounds their difficulties in processing—listening and decoding—what they hear.

From my point of view, the primary impairment in developmentally aphasic children is a deficiency in *central auditory processing*. The impairment is, in effect, a *central auditory disorder* (CAD), which produces "deficiencies in the ability to perceive sounds of speech categorically, to analyze and code speech in terms of a phonetic feature code, and to appreciate and utilize contextual information" (Eimas, 1979).

In some instances, aphasic children appear to be deaf because they stop listening to spoken language, since to them it seems like a nondecodable flow of human sounds. They may generalize this impairment by also ceasing to listen to environmental sounds, to animal and mechanical noises that they are able to decode. This may be a result of punishment by their parents, who do not understand how a child can hear nonhuman sounds but not respond to their speech.* See Eisenson (1985a) for a detailed consideration of central auditory deficiency as the basic impairment in developmental asphasia.

Few children are likely to learn to speak unless they are spoken to by parents or other persons who are concerned about the result of the quality of their caregiving (*available and capable caregivers*). Loving the child goes a long way, but it is not enough to get a neonate involved in language behavior. Perhaps the best explanation of what a parent or other caregiver must be able and willing to do comes from deVilliers and deVilliers (1979):

> Mothers (and fathers too . . .) tailor the length and complexity of their utterances to the linguistic ability of their children. Mothers' speech to one- and two-year-olds consists of simple, grammatically correct, short sentences that refer to concrete objects and events. There are few references to the past and almost none to the future. Sentence intonation and stress are greatly exaggerated, and clear pauses appear between sentences. (p. 99)

This type and quality of language production—"mother-ese" and "father-ese"—will not overwhelm a child with a flow of incomprehensible utterances. Such utterances may be compared with the response of an adult traveling in a foreign country who is exposed to a spoken language never heard before.

If, despite appropriate speech behavior, despite acceptable quality of

---

*When I am confronted with this problem I explain to the parent the difference between the two hemispheres in the kind of sounds each hemisphere normally processes. I emphasize that almost always the left hemisphere is the one that deals with spoken language; the right with nonspeech sounds.

physical and emotional care by the parents, and despite the absence of hearing loss or of evident mental retardation, the child fails to acquire language, we must look for other causes to explain the problem.

NEUROLOGICAL FINDINGS IN THE DEVELOPMENTALLY APHASIC

Brain Difference vs. Brain Pathology

As Geschwind (1979, p. 148) observed, "brains which show no pathology in the usual sense of the term may yet deviate from the normal." These brains differ in rates of development, either throughout the brain or in specific areas only. Such deviations, if they involve the parts of the brain that process language intake and output may account for some instances of severe language delay in children who are identified as aphasic or dysphasic.

Except for the severity of their language delay, many developmentally aphasic children do not present clear-cut "hard sign" evidence of central nervous system pathology. I include in "hard sign" evidence such defects as motor disabilities, sensory dysfunctions, and perceptual–motor delays or integrative impairments. Indicators in these categories are found in about one-third of the population who are behaviorally aphasic. Many more show evidence of at least "minimal brain dysfunction." Signs include delayed laterality, late walking, awkwardness, attention difficulties, and perceptual–motor irregularities. But some aphasic children, except for their severe delay in the comprehension and production of language, show neither the expected hard signs of neuropathology nor the more frequent "soft signs." However, as Ferry (1981) argues:

> Delay or deviation in language development is due to disordered brain function. . . . Speech and language delay or impairment may be the only symptom or sign of neurological impairment. This is a reflection of functional localization in which severe damage to a circumscribed area may occur while other areas of the brain remain perfectly intact. Thus, although a child with delayed speech development may have a perfectly normal general neurological examination, this should not rule out the possibility that his delayed speech is due to a neurological problem. (pp. 5–6)

Electroencephalographic (EEG) and related findings and other hard sign evidence of neuropathologies in children with severe language delay and/or disorder are reviewed in Eisenson (1984a, Chapter 5). These include studies by Forrest, Eisenson, and Stark (1967) who found that 37 of 73 children had abnormal EEGs and one by Rapin and Wilson (1978). The latter-named investigators found that in a population of 87 children considered to have structural brain damage based on neurological observation, 26 showed enlargement of the left temporal horn, 6 showed enlargement of the right temporal horn, and 14 showed enlargement of both left and right temporal horns. Rapin and Wilson note that "the lateral temporal cortex is concerned with auditory processing, and the left hemisphere with linguistic processing."

The implications of these findings are consistent with those of Luria (1982) and Geschwind (1979) and the general agreement among neuropsychologists and neurolinguists that the left temporal cortex has a special responsibility for the processing of speech signals. An impairment in this processing results in a disability to decode spoken language at the rate and quantity at which speech is usually presented. This, I believe, is the essence of developmental aphasia.

PERCEPTUAL DYSFUNCTIONS

During the mid 1960s to early 1970s, Eisenson and several colleagues conducted a series of studies on perceptual functioning in which they compared aphasic and postaphasic (dysphasic) children with normal peers. These studies are reviewed by Eisenson (1984a, Chapter 5). In the late 1970s and early 1980s, Tallal and her associates conducted a series of studies in the United States and England on the discriminative and sequencing abilities of dysphasic children. These studies are reviewed by Eisenson (1984a, Chapter 5); Stark, Mellits, and Tallal (1983); Tallal (1985); and Tallal and Piercy (1978). The following list summarizes their findings:

1. Defects (errors and delays) in the discrimination and sequencing of auditory events occur when the interstimulus interval between events is less than 150 milliseconds.
2. Discrimination problems appear when the auditory events have rapidly changing features and are of short duration. (These are characteristic of speech.)
3. Speech production errors in imitative tasks are related to errors in perceptual functioning.
4. Errors for nonverbal events are similar to those for speech.
5. Discriminative judgments are generally more accurate when subjects are permitted to make immediate responses than when short delays are introduced. The short-delay periods presented no problems for normal speaking peers. This finding is interpreted as indicating defective storage and/or retrieval strategies for auditory (speech) events.

Articulatory Apraxia and Dyspraxia

A small percentage of children with developmental aphasia who have made considerable progress in language comprehension may continue to have difficulties in oral language production. Some may, in fact, be suffering from oral (articulatory) dyspraxia rather than aphasia. This impairment may also be congenital and occur as an associated problem. Less frequently, the dyspraxia and the more severe apraxia may be a discrete impairment and confused with expressive aphasia.

Congenital oral dyspraxias are impairments in the ability to produce voluntary movements of the muscles of the larynx, pharynx, tongue, lips, palate, and cheeks which are required for an intended sequence of speech. Oral apraxia implies severe impairment. If the comprehension of oral language is not initially impaired, the child has potentially good capacity to take in and decode spoken language but has difficulty in the "mechanics" of production—the expression of encoding. It is not surprising to find that some children will reduce or completely turn away from linguistic communication because for them, normal communicative interchange is not possible. Thus, it is important to make a distinction between congenital aphasic impairments that produce a primary difficulty in language decoding and motor (productive) impairments that may be associated with the aphasia or may be a separate disability. Articulatory apraxia and dyspraxia for speech are considered in some detail in Eisenson (1984a, Chapter 10).

DEVELOPMENTAL APHASIA AND CHILDHOOD AUTISM

Is childhood autism an extreme form of developmental aphasia or is it a separate syndrome with overlapping features and a different etiology? May some children suffer from both pathologies, as Cohen, Caparulo, and Schaywitz (1976) believe? Is it more tenable to view the two as related syndromes and thus permit designations such as *aphasia with secondary autistic reactions* or *autism with aphasic components*? Because of our limited knowledge of the etiology of childhood autism, it is not possible to make a firm differential diagnosis based on organic causes. However, if we emphasize the cognitive and linguistic behaviors as the essential differential factors, we could make a case for a continuum of degrees of severity or for overlapping aberrant behaviors.

My own observations and reviews of clinical histories also suggest the possibility that misdiagnoses and consequent inappropriate treatment of children with developmental aphasia are conducive to producing withdrawal and other autistic expressions. In effect, the diagnosis produces the effects which in turn "justifies" the diagnosis. In comparing developmentally aphasic to autistic children, we need also take into account the presence in some autistic children of exceptional skills, such as verbal reproduction, arithmetic computation, "calendar minds," musical ability, and often remarkably proficient visuospatial orientation.

CHILDHOOD ACQUIRED
APHASIA

As indicated earlier in this chapter, the term *childhood acquired aphasia* should be restricted to children who had acquired language normally and then, as a result of identified cerebral pathology suffered through accident or disease, became impaired in previously established language functioning. For the sake of the present discussion, age 12 will be considered the upper limit of childhood. *Acquired dysphasia* is suggested as the appropriate term for residual or maintained deficits following a period of recovery.

How much impairment a given child experiences following the onset of involvement will vary considerably according to several factors, which include:

1. *Site and amount of brain lesion.* Acquired aphasia in children is more often associated with bilateral cerebral pathology than is the case with adults. Aphasic impairments also occur more often in children with right cerebral lesions than in adults.* However, "The risk of aphasia with right-brain injury, while higher in children than in adults, is still lower than the risk of aphasia following left-sided injury, regardless of age." (Satz & Bullard-Bates, 1981, p. 401).
2. *The degree of language at the onset of involvement.* This will vary considerably from child to child according to age at onset of impairment. We are more likely to find greater linguistic variability in 3 year olds than in those who are 10 or 11. What may constitute recovery for a 10 year old may be initial language acquisition for a normal 3 year old. Precocious children may have more to lose and more to regain than a slow or even normal 3-year-old child.
3. *Intelligence, sex, motivation, and stimulation.* These are additional factors that may acount for recovery and variability in early stages of recovery.

Causes

The etiology of aphasia in children is more likely to be associated with injury rather than with the vascular pathologies more frequent in adults. However, though rare, comparable vascular lesions do occur in children. (Literature on this subject is reviewed by Satz & Bullard-Bates, 1981, p. 400.) Neoplasms are the least likely cerebral pathology.

---

*This may be so because in young children, especially those who are below age 5, cerebral dominance for language may not be completely lateralized.

Patterns of Early Language Impairments

A striking and frequent feature of the early stage of acquired aphasia is *mutism*, the "loss of initiation of speech or more generally of the inability to communicate" (Hécaen, 1976). Many children, especially in the early acute stage, have great difficulty in auditory (verbal) comprehension. Fortunately, this impairment is of short duration. Hécaen (1976) also observes that "disturbances of naming have a still greater frequency and tend to persist, the lexical poverty being noted at later stages and even mentioned in school reports." On the motor-expressive side, articulatory impairments (dysarthrias) are frequently present in the early stages and are sometimes persistent. In Hécaen's longitudinal study, 4 of 12 cases had chronic dysarthrias.

Written Language Impairments

Among school age children with acquired aphasia, we are likely to find disturbances in previously established abilities for reading and writing. In most cases, there is a considerable way to go toward "complete" recovery. Hécaen reported that in his 1976 longitudinal study of 15 children, 3 children had persistent deficits in reading and 7 had deficits in writing. Table 9.1 sums up Hécaen's findings. Not included on the table is the relatively high incidence of arithmetic deficits. Hécaen found that 11 of the 15 cases in his study had such deficits.

A general finding of investigators of persistent deficits associated with acquired aphasia in children is that "even in cases of recovery from

Table 9.1. Frequency of Different Aphasic Symptoms in 15 Cases
Due to Left Hemisphere Lesions

	Number of Cases	Percentage	Evolution
Mutism	9	60	From 5 days to 3 months
Articulatory disorders	12	80	Persistent in 4 cases
Auditory verbal compre- hension disorders	6	40	Persistent in 1 case
Naming disorders	7	46	Persistent in 3 cases
Paraphasia	1	7	Disappearance
Reading disorders	9	60	Persistent in 3 cases
Writing disorders	13	86	Persistent in 7 cases

Note. From "Acquired Aphasia in Children and the Ontogenesis of Hemispheric Specializatoin in Children" by H. Hécaen, 1976, *Brain and Language, 3,* p. 124. Copyright 1982 by Academic Press. Used with permission.

aphasia, serious cognitive and academic sequelae were found'' (Satz & Bullard-Bates, 1981, p. 421).

For reviews of the literature on spoken and written deficits and cognitive impairments see Eisenson (1984a, Chapter 11) and Satz and Bullard-Bates (1981).

Chapter 10
Where to Go for
Professional Help

As indicated earlier, children with speech and/or language disorders, as well as those with hearing impairments, often require professional attention. Sometimes, the attention may consist of advice to parents on whether the presenting problem is merely a normal, developmental aspect of language and speech acquisition, which would improve in time. At other times, the advice might recommend early intervention. Routinely, presenting problems that have or may have a physical basis, such as cleft palate, laryngeal pathology, hearing loss, or neurological impairments must have medical clearance before speech or language therapy is undertaken. Medical clearance is also a *must* for all cases of voice problems.

In the United States and Canada, professional persons who are concerned with speech and language problems are usually identified as *speech–language pathologists*. Some may prefer to use the term *clinician* rather than *pathologist*; still others are called *speech therapists*. Those professionals who work with children or adults with hearing impairments are usually identified as *audiologists*. Those who work in educational settings and are responsible for the education and related needs of the deaf are known as *educators of the deaf.*

Many, perhaps most, professional persons who are specifically concerned with the diagnosis and treatment of speech, language, and hearing (communicative) disorders are members of the American Speech-Language-Hearing Association (ASHA).* In Canada, they are also likely to be members of the Canadian Speech and Hearing Association.

Although membership in ASHA alone is not a guarantee of professional competence, their certificates of clinical competence are awarded only to

---

*Membership in the American Speech-Language-Hearing Association is not limited to residents of the United States. ASHA members include citizens of Canada, Great Britian, Australia, New Zealand, and more than 30 other nations.

members whose qualifications include appropriate education, supervised clinical experience, and passing necessary examinations.

At the present time (1986) 46 state organizations in the United States have been approved by ASHA. About a third of the states require licensing, based on examinations, for persons who work with children who have speech-language or hearing disorders. Usually, the licensing requirements resemble those for the ASHA's Certificates of Clinical Competence. A referring professional or parent may find out from the state organization or from ASHA* whether licensing is required in a given state and the names of those who are licensed.

In addition to the United States and Canada, many countries have professional associations that serve functions similar to the American Speech–Language–Hearing Association and the Canadian Speech and Hearing Association. In Great Britain and Australia, Colleges of Speech Therapy provide both education and certification for professional speech and hearing clinicians (speech-language pathologists and audiologists). In several European countries, medical persons practice *phoniatrics*; nonmedical specialists practice *logopedics.*

Many state and municipal colleges and universities as well as private institutions have departments that provide professional help for children with communicative problems. Common names for such departments are Speech Pathology and Audiology, Speech and Hearing Disorders, or Communication Disorders. These departments may also have listings of certified or licensed practitioners in their regions. Most schools provide services through the secondary grades. Medical centers, both public and private, may also provide such services.

I would like to restate one point emphatically. Children, and adults as well, who have voice disorders or who in any way appear to have physical problems that may be associated with such symptoms should always be seen by a physician to determine whether medical treatment is needed before corrective therapy for speech, language, or hearing can be initiated. Continued consultation with the physician is highly desirable.

SELECTED RECOMMENDED READINGS

Since the 1960s, publication of research on normal and deviant speech and language acquisition in children has burgeoned. The research has been published in professional journals and more popular magazines, par-

---

*The address for ASHA is 10801 Rockville Pike, Rockville, MD, 20852. The address for the Canadian Speech and Hearing Association is 181 University Avenue, Toronto, Ontario, Canada M5H 3M7.

ticularly addressed to parents. Space limitation has necessitated leaving out writings that are equally deserving of inclusion. My selection is an attempt to include those that are authoritative but not weighted with an over-abundance of technical terminology. Many other publications, which are not included, undoubtedly meet these criteria. Interested readers will find references to such material in the few I selected under each heading.

Readings of General Interest

Eisenson, J., & Ogilvie, M. (1983). *Communicative disorders in children.* New York: Macmillan.   This book is an introductory textbook, intended for the beginner in the field of speech and language disorders. Because it employs a minimum of technical language, it is also appropriate for lay readers. The book emphasizes the roles of the classroom teacher and the parent in understanding and treating children with communicative problems.

Eisenson, J. (1975). *Is your child's speech normal?* Reading, MA: Addison-Wesley.   A brief and nontechnical explanation of normal speech and language acquisition and problems that could impair communication. It explains what parents and other concerned adults can do to help the child.

Language Acquisition and Language Delay

de Villiers, P. A., & de Villiers, J. G. (1979). *Early language.* Cambridge, MA: Harvard University Press.   A charming and sometimes amusing explanation of how children learn to speak and to understand language. The book considers the constraints of intelligence and conditions, such as deafness and dysphasia, on language acquisition.

Hopper, R. & Naremore, R. J. (1978). *Children's speech.* New York: Harper and Row.   The authors provide a practical introduction to the development of communicative abilities in children. Research literature is "translated" into lay terms.

Lewis, M. M. (1959). *Infant speech.* New York: Basic Books.   This book, which I consider a classic, is by a British expert who presents scholarly but readily understandable explanations of how children learn to talk. (Original work published in 1951 by Humanities Press.)

Stuttering and Cluttering

Bloodstein, O. (1975). *A handbook on stuttering.* Chicago: National Easter Seal Society for Crippled Children and Adults.   This nontechnical book reviews the research to date on stuttering and appropriate therapy for the child who stutters. It makes the point that what sounds like stuttering may be an aspect of normal speech development.

Bluemel, C. S. (1957). *The riddle of stuttering.* Danville, IL: The Interstate Press.   Bluemel, a psychiatrist who specialized in the treatment of stutterers, explains the riddle of stuttering and provides a therapeutic answer to the riddle. Despite the date of publication, it is contemporary in its view.

Eisenson, J., & Ogilvie, M. (1983). "Stuttering." In *Communicative disorders in children.* New York: Macmillan.   This chapter deals with the school age child who may be stuttering. It emphasizes the distinction between normal hesitations and stuttering and cluttering. The treatment of the young stutterer, at home and in school, is considered in detail.

Johnson, W. (1961). *Stuttering and what you can do about it.* Minneapolis: University of Minnesota Press.   The author offers advice that is still sound on how to prevent stuttering in children and how to treat stuttering children, if it is too late for prevention.

Weiss, D. (1964). *Cluttering.* Englewood Cliffs, NJ: Prentice-Hall.   Weiss, a medical expert on speech problems, describes and explains cluttering, a disorder of "tangled" language, and its relation to stuttering. Weiss believed that most stuttering originated in cluttering. Suggestions for treatment are provided in this concise and clearly written book.

Voice

Because of my belief that most children's voice problems result from imitating their elders, several of the references are primarily intended for adults:

Boone, D. R. (1983). *The voice and voice therapy.* Englewood Cliffs, NJ: Prentice-Hall.   The third edition of this book provides a clear exposition on how voice is produced as well as techniques for improvement.

Eisenson, J. (1985). *Voice and diction: A program for improvement,* 5th edition. New York: Macmillan.   The first half of this book deals with the production and improvement of voice.

Greene, M. C. (1980). *The voice and its disorders.* Philadelphia: Lippincott.   Though somewhat technical, Greene provides clear and succinct explanations of the most frequent disorders of voice.

Wilson, D. K. (1979). *Voice problems of children.* Baltimore: Williams & Wilkins.   Although the discussion of children's voice problems is somewhat technical, the suggested exercises and therapy materials are easy to understand.

Wood, B. S. (1976). *Children and communication.* Englewood Cliffs, NJ: Prentice-Hall.   In the chapter on "The Child's Voice Communicates," the author explains that the voice is a powerful channel for communicating ideas, feelings, and attitudes, both obvious and subtle. Wood presents her views on how children learn to recognize meanings and feelings as they are expressed in adult vocal behavior and, in turn, how they learn to communicate their own thoughts and emotions in their messages. Conflict messages, ones in which the words are at variance with the voice, for example sarcasm and innuendo, are difficult for children under the age of 12 to understand and resolve.

Brain Different Children

Clements, S. D. (1966). *Minimal brain dysfunction in children.* NINDB Monograph 3. Washington, DC: U.S. Department of Health, Education, and Welfare.   This mongraph summed up the research, to the date of its publication, on children with "minimal brain damage." Though on the technical side, it is not difficult to understand.

Ludlow, C. L., & Doran-Quine, M. E. (Eds.). (1979.) *The neurological bases of language disorders in children: Methods and directions for research.* NINCDS Monograph 22. Bethesda, MD: U.S. Department of Health, Education, and Welfare.   The papers in this monograph were given at a symposium on the title subject. Topics include the relationship of the brain to language function, mother–child nonverbal communications, brain dominance related to language, how to study children's language behavior, and research needs for future study. This selection is technical, to be sure, but a must for persons who seek an in-depth understanding of the neurological bases of language and what may go wrong that impairs normal language acquisition.

References

American Psychiatric Association. (1980). *Diagnostic and statistical manual of mental disorders* (3rd ed.). Washington, DC.

Andrews, G., Craig, A., Feyer, A., Hoddinott, S., Howie, P., & Nielson, M. (1983). Stuttering: A review of research findings and theories,circa 1982. *Journal of Speech and Hearing Disorders, 48,* 226–246.

Anthony, D. & Associates. (1971). *Seeing essential English.* Anaheim, CA: Anaheim Union School District.

Benton, A. (1978). The cognitive functioning of children with developmental dysphasia. In M. Wyke (Ed.), *Developmental dysphasia.* New York: Academic Press.

Berko-Gleason, J. (1983). Otitis media and language development. *Pediatrics, 71,* 644–645.

Boone, D. R. (1983). *The voice and voice therapy,* (3rd ed.). Englewood Cliffs, NJ: Prentice-Hall.

Bornstein, H., Hamilton, K., Sauliner, K., & Roy, H. (1975). *The signed English dictionary for preschool and elementary levels.* Washington, DC: Gallaudet College.

Bosma, J. F. (1975). Anatomic and physiologic development of the speech apparatus. In D. B. Tower (Ed.), *The nervous system: Vol. 3., Human communication and its disorders.* New York: Raven Press.

Bowlby, J. (1958). The nature of the child's tie to the mother. *International Journal of Psychoanalysis, 39,* 350–373.

Bruner, J. (1975). The ontogenesis of speech acts. *Journal of Child Language, 2,* 1–19.

Bzock, K. R., & League, R. (1971). *Receptive–Expressive Emergent Language Scale (REEL).* Baltimore: University Park Press.

Canadian Minister of National Health and Welfare. (1984). *Childhood hearing impairment.* Ottawa, Canada: National Health and Welfare Service, Health Service Directorate.

Carrow-Woolfolk, E., & Lynch, J. L. (1982). *An integrative approach to language disorders in children.* New York: Grune and Stratton.

Coplon, J. (1983). *The Early Language Milestone (ELM) Scale.* Tulsa, OK: Modern Education Corporation.

Cohen, D. J., Caparulo, B. S., & Schaywitz, B. (1976). Primary childhood aphasia and childhood autism. *Journal of the Academy of Child Psychiatry, 15,* 604–644.

Damasio, A. (1981). The nature of aphasia: signs and syndromes. In M. T. Sarno (Ed.), *Acquired aphasia.* New York: Academic Press.

Davis, H., & Silverman, S. R. (1978). *Hearing and deafness.* New York: Holt, Rinehart, and Winston.

Davis, J. M., & Hardick, E. J. (1981). *Rehabilitative audiology for children and adults.* New York: John Wiley.

de Villiers, P. A., & de Villiers, J. G. (1979). *Early Language.* Cambridge, MA: Harvard University Press.

127

Downs, M. (1983). Audiologist's overview of sequelae of early otitis media. *Pediatrics, 71*, 643–644.

Eimas, P. D. (1979). On the processing of speech: Some implications for language development. In C. L. Ludlow, and M. E. Doran-Quine (Eds.), *Neurological bases of language disorders in children*. NINCDS. Monograph No. 22. Washington, DC: U. S. Department of Health, Education, and Welfare.

Eisenson, J. (Ed.). (1975). *Stuttering: A second symposium*. New York: Harper and Row.

Eisenson, J. (1984a). *Aphasia and related disorders in children*. New York: Harper and Row.

Eisenson, J. (1984b). *Reading for meaning*. Tulsa, OK: Modern Education Corporation.

Eisenson, J. (1985a). Central auditory disorders and developmental aphasia. *Human Communication Canada, 9*, 13–16.

Eisenson, J. (1985b). *Voice and diction: A program for improvement* (5th ed.). New York: Macmillan.

Eisenson, J., & Ogilvie, M. (1983). *Communicative disorders in children*. New York: Macmillan.

Fay, W. H., & Schuler, A. L. (1980). *Emerging language in autistic children*. Baltimore: University Park Press.

Ferry, P. C. (1981). Neurological considerations in children with learning disabilities. In R. W. Keith (Ed.), *Central auditory and language disorders in children*. San Diego, CA: College-Hill Press.

Forrest, T., Eisenson, J., & Stark, J. (1967). EEG findings in 113 nonverbal children. Abstract in *Electroencephalographic Clinical Neuropsychology, 22*, 291.

Freeman, B. J., & Ritvo, E. R. (1977). In J. Budde (Ed.), *Advocacy and autism*. Lawrence, KS: University of Kansas Press.

Furth, H. (1966). *Thinking without language*. New York: Free Press.

Garrard, K. R., & Clark, B. S. (1984). Otitis media: The role of speech-language pathologists. *ASHA, 27*, 35–40.

Geschwind, N. (1979). Anatomical foundations of language and dominance. In C. L. Ludlow & M. E. Doran-Quine (Eds.), *The neurological bases of language disorders in children*. NINCDS Monograph No. 22. Washington, DC: U. S. Department of Health, Education, and Welfare.

Ginsberg, I. A., & White, T. P. (1978). Otological considerations of audiology. In J. Katz (Ed.), *Handbook of clinical audiology* (2nd ed.). Baltimore: Williams and Wilkins.

Greene, M. C. (1980). *The voice and its disorders* (4th ed.). Philadelphia: Lippincott.

Gustason, G., Pfetzinger, D., & Aswolkow, E. (1972). *Signing exact English*. Rossmoor, CA: Modern Signs Press.

Halliday, M. A. K. (1975). *Learning how to mean*. London: Edward Arnold.

Hécaen, H. (1976). Acquired aphasia in children and the ontogenesis of hemispheric functional specialization. *Brain and Language, 3*, 114–134.

Holzman, M. (1983). *The language of children*. Englewood Cliffs, NJ: Prentice-Hall.

Hopper, R., & Naremore, R. J. (1978). *Children's speech*. New York: Harper and Row.

Howie, P. M. (1976). The identification of genetic components in speech disorders. *Australian Journal of Human Communication Disorders, 4*, 155–163.

Ingram, D. (1977). *Phonological disability in children*. New York: Elsevier.

Kanner, L. (1943). Autistic disturbances of affective contact. *Nervous child, 2*, 217–250.

Karelitz, K., & Fischelli, V. R. (1962). The cry thresholds of normal infants and those with brain damage. *Journal of Pediatrics, 61* (5), 679–685.

Kidd, K. K. (1980). Genetic models of stuttering. *Journal of Fluency Disorders, 5*, 187–201.

Kinsbourne, M. & Caplan, P. J. (1979). *Children's learning and attention problems*. Boston: Little, Brown.

Lewis, M. M. (1959). *Infant speech*. New York: Humanities Press. (Original work published in 1951 by Humanities Press.)

Lieberman, P. (1966). *Intonation, perception, and language*. Cambridge, MA: MIT Press.

Lillywhite, H. S., & Bradley, D. P. (1969). *Communication problems in mental retardation*. New York: Harper and Row.

Ling, D. (1976). *Speech and the hearing impaired child*. Washington, DC: Alexander Graham Bell Association for the Deaf.

Luper, H. L., & Ford, S. C. (1980). Disorders of fluency. In R. J. Van Hattum (Ed.), *Communication disorders*. New York: Macmillan.

Luria, A. R. (1982). *Language and cognition*. Washington, DC: V. H. Winston.

Martin, F. N. (1986). *Introduction to audiology* (3rd ed.). Englewood Cliffs, NJ: Prentice-Hall.

Maskarinec, A. S., Cairns, G. F., Butterfield, E. C., Weamer, L. K. (1981). Longitudinal observations of individual infant's vocalizations. *Journal of Speech and Hearing Disorders, 46*, 267–273.

Mecham, M. J., Jex, L., & Jones, J. D. (1967). *Utah Test of Language Development*. Salt Lake City: Communication Research Associates, Inc.

Menyuk, P., & Looney, P. L. (1972). Relationships among components of the grammar in language disorders. *Journal of Speech and Hearing Research, 15*, 395–406.

Miller, J. F., & Yoder, D. E. (1974). An ontogenetic language teaching strategy for retarded children. In R. L. Schiefelbusch and L. L. Lloyd (Eds.), *Language perspectives, retardation, and intervention*. Baltimore: University Park Press.

Murry, T., & Murry, J. (Eds.). (1980). *Infant communication: Cry and early speech*. San Diego, CA: College-Hill Press.

Newby, H., & Popelka, G. (1985). *Audiology* (5th ed.). Englewood Cliffs, NJ: Prentice-Hall.

Northern, J. L. (1984). *Hearing disorders*. Boston: Little Brown.

Ostwald, P. F., & Peltzman, P. (1974). The cry of the human infant. *Scientific American, 230*, 84–90.

Perkins, W. H. (1977). *Speech pathology* (2nd ed.). St. Louis: Mosby.

Piggot, L. R. (1979). Overview of selected basic research in autism. *Journal of Autism and Developmental Disabilities, 9*, 199–218.

Prizant, B. M. (1983). Language acquisition and communicative behavior in autism. *Journal of Speech and Hearing Disorders, 48*, 296–307.

Rapin, I., & Wilson, B. C. (1978). Children with developmental language disability. In M. A. Wyke (Ed.), *Developmental dysphasia*. New York: Academic Press.

Renfrew, C., & Murphy, K. (1964). *The child who does not talk*. London: Heinemann.

Ross, A. O. (1980). *Psychological disorders of children* (2nd ed.). New York: McGraw-Hill.

Rutter, M. (1978). Diagnosis and definition of childhood autism. *Journal of Autism and Childhood Schizophrenia, 8*, 139–161.

Sander, E. K. (1972). When are speech sounds learned? *Journal of Speech and Hearing Disorders, 37*, 55–63.

Satz, P., & Bullard-Bates, C. (1981). Acquired aphasia in children. In M. T. Sarno (Ed.), *Acquired aphasia*. New York: Academic Press.

Schuler, A. L. (1984). Childhood autism. In J. Eisenson, *Aphasia and related disorders in children*. New York: Harper and Row.

Shriberg, L. D. (1980). Developmental phonological disorders. In T. S. Hixon, L. D. Shriberg, & J. H. Saxman (Eds.), *Introduction to communicative disorders*. Englewood Cliffs, NJ: Prentice-Hall.

Silverman, S. R., Lane, H. S., & Calvert, D. R. (1978). Early and elementary education. In H. Davis and S. R. Silverman, *Hearing and deafness*. New York: Holt, Rinehart, and Winston.

Stark, R. E., Mellits, E. D., & Tallal, P. (1983). Behavioral attributes of speech and language disorders. In C. L. Ludlow, & J. A. Cooper, (Eds.), *Genetic aspects of speech and language disorders*. New York: Academic Press.

Stemach, G., & Eisenson, J. (1977). *Language sampling with stuttering children*. Unpublished paper, Institute for Childhood Aphasia, San Francisco State University.

Stocker, B. (1976). *The Stocker probe technique*. Tulsa, OK: Modern Education Corporation.

Strome, M. (1982). Common laryngeal disorders in children. In M. D. Filte (Ed.), *Phoniatry voice disorders in children*. Springfield, IL: Charles C Thomas.

Tallal, P. (1985). Neuropsychological research approaches to the study of central auditory processing. *Human Communication Canada, 9*, 17–22.

Tallal, P., & Piercy, M. (1978). Defects of auditory perception. In M. A. Wyke (Ed.), *Developmental dysphasia*. New York: Academic Press.

Truby, H. M., Bosma, J. F., & Lind, J. (1966). *Newborn infant cry*. Uppsala, Sweden: Almquist and Wiksells.

Van Riper, C. (1971). *The nature of stuttering*. Englewood Cliffs, NJ: Prentice Hall. (2nd ed., 1982.)

Van Riper, C., & Emerick, L. (1984). *Speech correction* (7th ed.). Englewood Cliffs, NJ: Prentice-Hall.

Wasz-Hockert, O., Lind, J., Vuorenkoski, V., Partanen, T., & Valanne, E. (1968). The infant cry. In *Clinics in developmental medicine*, No. 29. London: Spastics International Medical Publications.

Weiss, D. (1964). *Cluttering*. Englewood Cliffs, NJ: Prentice-Hall.

Weissbluth, M. (1984). *Cry babies*. New York: Arbor House.

West, R. (1958). An agnostic's speculations about stuttering. In J. Eisenson (Ed.), *Stuttering: A symposium*. New York: Harper and Row.

Wilson, D. K. (1979). *Voice problems in children* (2nd ed). Baltimore: Williams and Wilkins.

Wolff, P. H. (1966). The natural history of crying and other vocalizations in early infancy. In B. M. Foss (Ed.), *Determinants of infant behavior* (vol. 4.). London: Methuen.

Author Index

131

Subject Index

About the Author

Jon Eisenson, a Diplomate in Clinical Psychology (American Board of Examiners in Professional Psychology) is widely known as a psychologist who specializes in the research and treatment of children and adults with language and speech problems. He is an Emeritus Professor of Hearing and Speech Science, Stanford University, and a former Distinguished Professor of Special Education, San Francisco State University. He was director of programs for the study of aphasic children at Stanford and San Francisco State Universities and, before coming to California, Director of the Queens College (City University of New York) Speech and Hearing Clinic.

Dr. Eisenson served on the faculties of Brooklyn College, the College of Physicians and Surgeons (Columbia University) and as a visiting professor at other universities in the United States, Australia, and Israel. He is the author of numerous articles and textbooks on the psychology of language, communication disorders, and on acquired and congenital aphasia. As a hobby, he writes and has published verses for children. The most recent is *My Special Zoo.*

Psychology Practitioner Guidebooks

Editors
Arnold P. Goldstein, Syracuse University
Leonard Krasner, SUNY at Stony Brook
Sol L. Garfield, Washington University

Elsie M. Pinkston & Nathan L. Linsk—CARE OF THE ELDERLY:
A Family Approach

Donald Meichenbaum—STRESS INOCULATION TRAINING

Sebastiano Santostefano—COGNITIVE CONTROL THERAPY
WITH CHILDREN AND ADOLESCENTS

Lillie Weiss, Melanie Katzman & Sharlene Wolchik—TREATING
BULIMIA: A Psychoeducational Approach

Edward B. Blanchard & Frank Andrasik—MANAGEMENT OF
CHRONIC HEADACHES: A Psychological Approach

Raymond G. Romanczyk—CLINICAL UTILIZATION OF
MICROCOMPUTER TECHNOLOGY

Philip H. Bornstein & Marcy T. Bornstein—MARITAL THERAPY:
A Behavioral-Communications Approach

Michael T. Nietzel & Ronald C. Dillehay—PSYCHOLOGICAL
CONSULTATION IN THE COURTROOM

Elizabeth B. Yost, Larry E. Beutler, M. Anne Corbishley & James R.
Allender—GROUP COGNITIVE THERAPY: A Treatment
Approach for Depressed Older Adults

Lillie Weiss—DREAM ANALYSIS IN PSYCHOTHERAPY

Edward A. Kirby & Liam K. Grimley—UNDERSTANDING AND
TREATING ATTENTION DEFICIT DISORDER

Jon Eisenson—LANGUAGE AND SPEECH DISORDERS
IN CHILDREN

Eva L. Feindler & Randolph B. Ecton—ADOLESCENT ANGER
CONTROL: Cognitive-Behavioral Techniques

Michael C. Roberts—PEDIATRIC PSYCHOLOGY: Psychological
Interventions and Strategies for Pediatric Problems

Daniel S. Kirschenbaum, William G. Johnson & Peter M. Stalonas, Jr.—
TREATING CHILDHOOD AND ADOLESCENT OBESITY

W. Stewart Agras—EATING DISORDERS: Management of Obesity,
Bulimia and Anorexia Nervosa